SUPER *Virility*

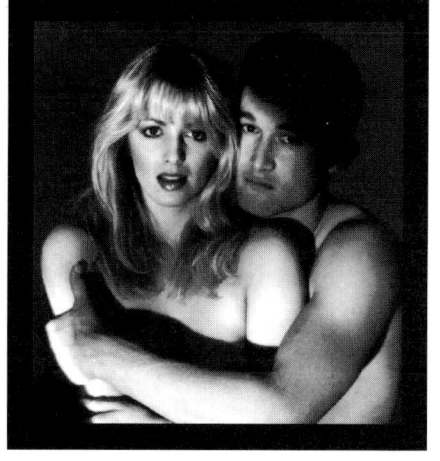

THE ULTIMATE GUIDE TO SEXUAL HAPPINESS

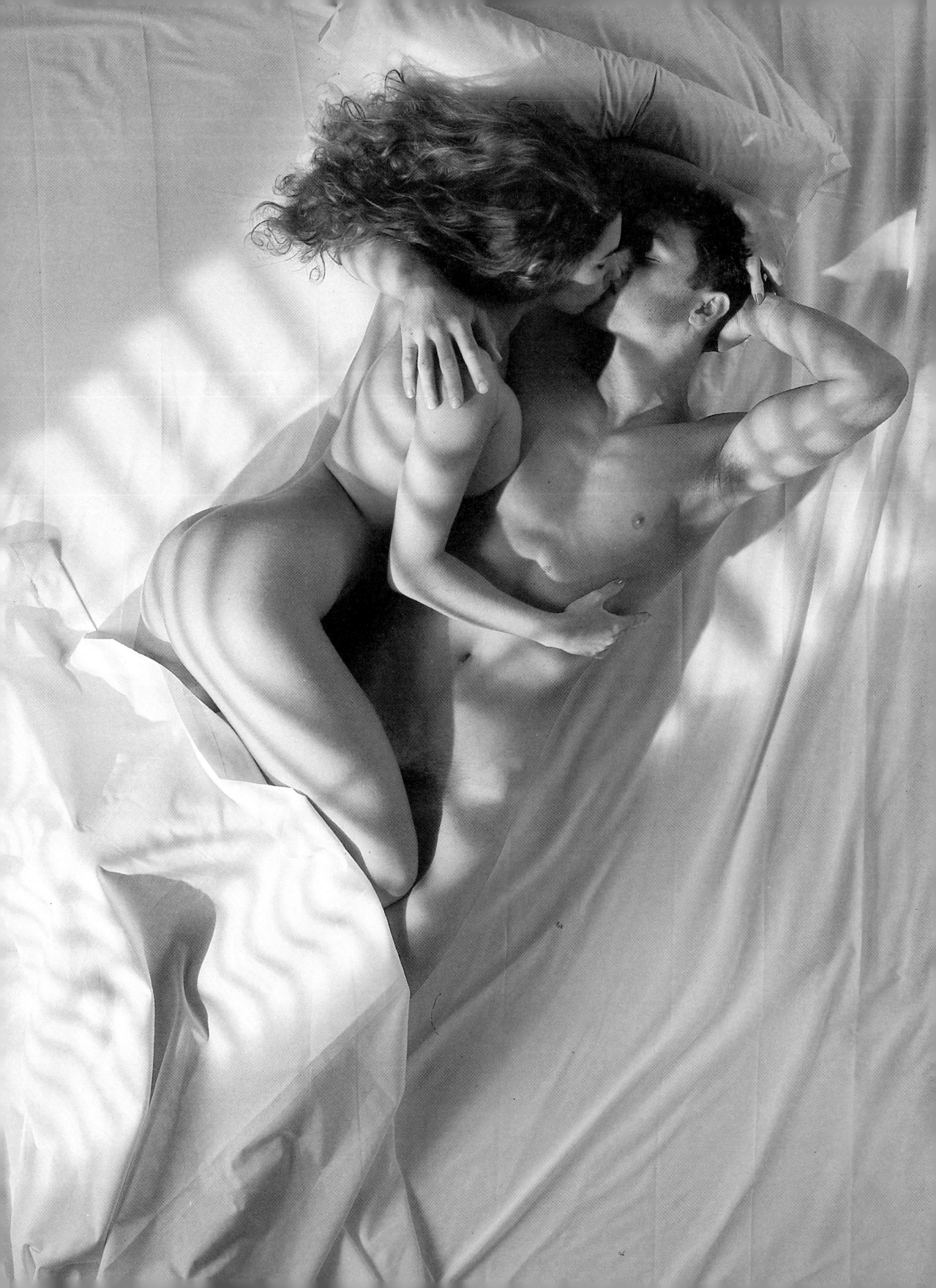

SUPER *Virility*

THE ULTIMATE GUIDE TO SEXUAL HAPPINESS

Susan Quilliam &
Ian Grove-Stephensen

ANAYA
PUBLISHERS LTD

First published in Great Britain in 1992 by Anaya Publishers Ltd, Strode House,
44-50 Osnaburgh Street, London NW1 3ND

Text copyright © Transformation Management Ltd 1992

The authors hereby assert to the publishers and their licensees their moral right
to be identified as the Authors of the Work

Design: Phil Marritt

Photographs:
© Zefa: pages 12-13, 17, 25, 28, 31, 32, 37, 39, 40, 42, 44, 47, 54, 64, 66, 68,
73, 74, 75, 76-7, 78-9, 83, 88, 90, 91, 92, 96, 101, 102, 104, 112, 114,
120-1, 126, 131, 136, 141, 142, 144-5, 152, 154.
© Marshall Cavendish Ltd: jacket; pages 1, 2, 8, 18-19, 20, 21, 52-3, 58-9,
63, 80-1, 94, 106-7, 109, 118-9, 124, 135, 136, 147, 149.
Reproduced with permission from the books *The Loving Touch*, *The Sensual Touch*,
The Intimate Touch, *The Personal Touch* and from the partwork *Face to Face*.

All rights reserved.
No part of this publication may be reproduced, stored in
a retrieval system, or transmitted, in any form or by
any means, electronic, mechanical, photocopying,
recording or otherwise, without the permission of the
copyright holder.

British Library Cataloguing in Publication Data
Quilliam, Susan
Supervirility: The ultimate guide to sexual happiness.
I. Title II. Grove-Stephensen, Ian
613.9081

ISBN 1-85470-080-4

Typeset by Marritt Associates

Printed and bound by Butler and Tanner Ltd, Frome and London

Contents

ACKNOWLEDGEMENTS 7

INTRODUCTION 8

Supervirility – our sexual birthright ● The barrier of fear ● The real facts
Supervirility – the challenge ● What this book does, and how
Your personalized action plan

PART I - BODY SUPERVIRILITY

1 Your body, your sexuality 20
The guided tour ● The private parts ● When you get aroused ● When blocks arise

2 Building your body 28
Food for love ● Sexual supplements ● Stimulating stimulants
Drink to me only ● Light my fire – or not ● What of drugs? ● Sleeping soundly
Relaxing for pleasure ● Keeping moving ● Action plan

3 Looking good and getting close 36
Looking good ● Dressing up ● Sounding good ● Getting close ● Moving together

4 When illness strikes 40
Bodyworks – not working ● When blood flow drops ● Brain power and nerve
nuisances ● When hormones fade ● Taking the tablets ● Sexual nasties

5 Body help 46
First checks ● Getting support ● Classes and courses
Complementary help ● Traditional help

PART II - MIND SUPERVIRILITY

6 Breaking free of the past 54
Past influences ● Tracking down the messages ● The essential contradiction
Where are you now? ● When the past hooks you ● Breaking free

7 Sexual myths 64
The myths ● A real man ● A real woman ● Real sex ● Debunking the myths

8 Coping with stress 68
Finding the balance ● Assessing your stress level ● Taking action

9 Building a Supervirile personality 74
Feeling good about yourself ● Being open to requests ● Asking for what you want
Relaxing into intimacy ● Feeling the emotions ● Letting pleasure take you over
Shrugging off problems ● Introducing innovations ● Celebrating success

Part III - Relationship Supervirility

10 Understanding your partner 82
Your partner's past • Life changes • Sexual mismatches • Finding out

11 When your love blocks your lust 88
What underlies your relationship? • Where are you now? • Bridging the gap

12 Building a Supervirile relationship 96
Clearing the past • Avoiding overdependency • Reducing rage
Developing trust • Contacting feelings • Talking it through
Problem solving • Setting goals • Checking progress

13 Other options 102
Erotica • Prostitutes • Having an affair • Doing without sex

Part IV - Sexual Supervirility

14 Her body, her sexuality 108
Her body • Her arousal • Her blocks • How the mismatch works
The good news • Comparing notes

15 First moves 114
Setting the scene • Aphrodisiacs – or not? • Erotic thoughts • Sounds and words

16 Sensual touching 118
Undressing and after • Massage hints • Sensuous exploration

17 On your own 124
Starting off • Moving on

18 Getting it up 130
Showing her how • Her turn

19 Pleasure without penetration 136
Her pleasure • Joining in • Your pleasure together

20 Pleasure with penetration 140
Preparing for penetration • Entering in

21 Orgasm 148
Tipping over the edge • Holding back • Helping her on
Coming together • Afterwards

Last words 154

Appendix A Getting outside help 155
Possibilities • What do you do in counselling? • Making it work

Appendix B Resources 158
Resources in the UK • International organisations

Appendix C Further Reading 159

ACKNOWLEDGEMENTS

One of the last great taboos is to talk or, even worse, to write about the fact that not all of us, all the time, are able to have the sex life of our dreams. Contrary to all myths, all changing-room tales and all media hype, sometimes our desire for sex dies or our ability to fulfil our desire fades.

So we are delighted to have the opportunity to write *Supervirility,* which we hope not only tackles the issue head on, but in the process debunks myths, offers reassurance and, on some occasions, tells the truth about sexuality for the first time. We aim not only to break the taboo and admit the problem, but also to offer hope that it is possible not only to have Supervirility but to claim it back even after it has temporarily faded away.

The book has been compiled from a number of sources: academic, medical and pragmatic. We have chosen not to continuously weight down the text with references to these, but we would like to thank here the wide range of people who have given us inspiration and support.

We have gratefully drawn on insights from the founders of sex therapy, who have over the last two decades transformed society's ideas of what is possible in an intimate relationship: people such as Alex Comfort, Helen Singer-Kaplan, Alfred Kinsey, William Masters and Virginia Johnson. We thank them for their continuing inspiration.

We have equally gratefully drawn from other sources in the field of psychology: humanistic psychology strands such as Co-counselling and TA (Transactional Analysis); more recent developments such as hypnotherapy and NLP (Neuro-Linguistic Programming). To the gurus of these schools, Richard Bandler, Eric Berne, Milton Erickson, John Grinder and Harvey Jackins, we also offer thanks.

Several specialist consultants helped us in a variety of ways, inspiring and supporting us, through their writings or their face-to-face meetings, to develop the arguments of the book. Our special thanks go to Dr John Bancroft, Dr Malcom Carruthers of the Positive Health Centre, Dr Martin Cole, Anne Dixon, Windy Dryden, Dr Gingel of Southmead Hospital, Judi Hildebrand of the Institute of Family Therapy, Val Hill of Brook Advisory Centres, Nikki Henriques, Sandra Leiblum and Raymon D. Rosen, Dr John Moran and Sue Pallenburg of the London Institute of Human Sexuality, James Nichol, Dr M. J. Pryor of St Peter's Hospital, Jane Ridley of the Maudsley Hospital, Deirdre Sanders, Gabriele Stutz.

Several organizations offered us contacts, information and support during our work. We would particularly like to thank: the Association of Sexual and Marital Therapists, the British Association of Counselling, the British Pregnancy Advisory Service, the Brook Advisory Centres, the Family Planning Association, the Institute of Sexual Education and Research, the Institute for Psychosexual Medicine, the London Institute for the Study of Human Sexuality, Survivors.

To Marj Thoburn and RELATE, formerly the National Marriage Guidance Council, our special thanks for allowing us to draw on their experience, their contacts and their friendly support.

Most especially, however, we would like to thank those people with experience of sex therapy and counselling who contributed to our research. Our discussions with them – men and women – gave us motivation and inspiration; their experiences informed the book on every level. To Bernard Collen, Martin and Joanna, and all the others who have asked not to be named, we give our heartfelt gratitude for their courage in sharing their experiences.

We would also like to mention all the people who have been involved in the making of the book. Barbara Levy, our agent, as always started the book off. Julia Howard, Felicity Sinclair and Jenni Tibble helped with the research and kept us organized on a day-to-day level; Julia transcribed discussions with her customary sensitivity.

At Anaya, Stan Remington, Carey Smith, Yvonne McFarlane, Melissa Henry, Karen Sullivan, Kay Hyman and designer Phil Marritt brought the book to its readers.

Finally, we would like to thank each other for all the help, support and love that has gone into the making of the book. We hope that it will give new insight and inspiration to everyone who wishes to have Supervirility.

**Ian Grove-Stephensen
and Susan Quilliam
1992**

INTRODUCTION

We all deserve good sex, for the whole of our lives.

For too many of us, however, good sex tends to get left behind as time passes. Just at the point where career, family life and general self-satisfaction start to come together, we find the whole thing being undermined by the fact that our sex lives are beginning to diminish.

Perhaps, physically, we begin to realize that we are less active than we were. Perhaps we start buying into the myth that sex drive inevitably drops as time passes. Perhaps, too, our relationship, though still full of love and contentment, has lost the spark of lust it had when we met. All these factors, and many others, are reflected in the slow but seemingly unstoppable decline in our enjoyment of sex.

For some of us, the problems are sudden and frightening. Perhaps one night, for the first time in our lives, we can't get an erection. We stifle the panic, but it stays with us, gnawing away with its thought of 'next time'. Perhaps we find that the quick, lustful acts of our earlier years are giving way to protracted sessions, where we may even wonder whether we are going to be able to come at all.

For many more of us, there are no crises, just a slow drop in quantity or quality. And in many ways that is far worse. We may have a creeping realization that, whereas this time last year we were making love three times a week, this time this year it is three times a month. Or we may have a slow awareness that love-making is still enjoyable, but sometimes... The word boredom is not one we would ever say out loud, but it is still there, unspoken, at the back of our minds.

Sex is vital to us, and so it should be. We have every right to demand that, however long lasting our relationship, sex be as enjoyable and exciting as it was at the start. In fact, we should even demand

INTRODUCTION

that it get more enjoyable and more fulfilling as time goes by. Suppose we started a new project, a job at work, a sport or a skill, and we were told that the more we practised it, the less we would enjoy it. Of course we would be horrified. In all areas of our lives, we expect to fulfil ourselves more, the more we practise; to get better at things as we grow older and wiser. Why shouldn't the same be true of sex?

SUPERVIRILITY – OUR SEXUAL BIRTHRIGHT

So what have we a right to expect, what have we a right to demand from sex, throughout our lives? We as authors think that everyone has a right to expect to:

- be a sexual person, whose appearance turns a partner on;

- have the basic energy for the act of sex;

- have a lasting desire to make love regularly;

- be confident of bypassing any sexual blocks;

- respond to a partner with deep emotion, affection and love;

- enjoy sex fully – by seeing, hearing, smelling, tasting and touching;

- improve love-making with thoughts, words and fantasies;

- be sexually active, through erection, movement, thrusting, touching, stroking, licking;

- relax and be made love to;

- give and get pleasure with abandonment;

- know the appropriate ways to help a partner towards orgasm and/or ejaculation;

- have orgasm and ejaculation easily and enjoyably;

- be able to let go after love-making; and

- be certain that all this is possible the next time round.

Perhaps this seems like a great deal to ask for. We are not only demanding sexuality, but supersexuality; not only virility, but *Supervirility*. Yet, surely such an easy and natural enjoyment of sex is what we all deserve. Because, in fact, we have all had the possibility of such enjoyment from the moment we were born.

THE BARRIER OF FEAR

So what stops us from having it all? What stops us from achieving Supervirility, here and now, at once?

Maybe our bodies have lost the edge they once had. Maybe mentally we have lost our capacity for sexual fulfilment. Maybe, with all the best intentions in the world, it is our relationship that is causing the blocks. Or maybe it is our sexual skill or technique that holds us back from Supervirility. In all these ways, we may be denying ourselves the sex we need and deserve. And, as time passes, we may begin to panic, as we see the possibility of good, regular sex slipping away.

The truth is, however, that all the above blocks – of body, mind, relationship or sexual skill – are removable. Not one is permanent, not one needs to stay in place, however long it has been there. It is never too late to reclaim sexuality, to overcome failing desire, to win out over the most challenging of sexual crises. And we can do more than that; we can move our love-making on, take up new ideas, try out new skills, continually enhance our sexuality.

The main block to achieving such sexual enhancement and maintaining it for the rest of our lives is, however, inside us. It is not boredom or illness or being trapped in our relationship. The main block is fear – based on the belief that, as time passes, we are bound to start to see our sexuality slipping away. For we are surrounded by messages that tell us that sex fades. From roadside posters; from page three of the tabloids; from our growing children; from our pensioner parents; even from self-help books (who should know better), we hear the message that sex is at its peak early in our lives and that, as time passes, we will naturally and inevitably slip into a less sexual partnership. All too often we accept that.

But, if we dare to contradict the myths, and to look closely and openly at our own sex lives, given the commitment and the courage to change, we can choose Supervirility for ourselves, here and now.

The first step in making this choice is to look at our fears, and meet them head on. In the course of compiling this book, we as authors asked a number of men what their views about lifelong sexuality were. The same fears emerged again and again, underpinning their attitudes to themselves and to their love-making. Here are typical ones.

'I suppose I've expected not to want it as much as time passes; so when I don't want it, I just go with that.'

'I'm terrified at the thought that one day I won't be able to get it up any more – or at any rate, whenever I want to...then I wouldn't feel like a real man.'

'I'm obviously not as attractive now as I was; I may get bald, put on weight, develop wrinkles. It's inevitable, and so are the effects on my sex life.'

'I worry that my orgasms are just going to get further and further apart.'

'Time passing means getting less sexual... that's the truth.'

These are real fears held by real people. No wonder that, when these fears come to our minds, we can get into a kind of panic spiral, where everything seems uncertain and the whole point of love-making is lost.

THE REAL FACTS

But are these fears realistic? Some are pure myth, and need to be debunked as quickly as possible. Some have an element of truth in them, so need to be clarified. Some are based on ignorance so may need new skills or knowledge added on as ballast.

Let's take a closer look at these fears:

The fear: 'I suppose I've expected not to want it as much as time passes; so when I don't want it, I go with that.'

The fact: If you buy into this, you are shortchanging yourself. The hard truth is that the first few months with the one you love had an edge of lust that you probably can't ever recapture unless you start again with a new partner. But once lust dies, other elements such as knowledge and experience take over and contain the possibility for sex to be actually much more exciting and fulfilling than it ever was in the days of your first fumble.

The fear: 'I'm terrified at the thought that, one day, I won't be able to get it up any more – or at any rate, whenever I want to...then I wouldn't feel like a real man.'

The fact: Not getting it up (or erectile difficulty, as it is called in the textbooks) can be physically or emotionally caused, and can strike at any time of life. The fact is that occasional erectile difficulty happens to most men – a study of pre-industrial societies showed that eighty per cent had 'magic cures' for impotence! But chronic erectile problems are caused more often than not by sheer panic that – guess what – you won't be able to get it up next time. As for not being a real man, as we show later in the book, a lack of erection never indicates a lack of masculinity – and a superhard erection is certainly no guarantee of Supervirility.

The fear: 'I'm obviously not as attractive now as I was; I may get bald, put on weight, develop wrinkles. It's inevitable, and so are the effects on my sex life.'

The fact: It is true that as we get older, physical changes do occur – though being young doesn't mean you necessarily avoid these; even men in their late teens may be bald, plump and wrinkled, have no energy or lose their stamina. Equally, you can do a great deal to stay looking attractive and healthy whatever your age. However, these facts miss the essential point: whatever the media claim, physical attractiveness is no sign of sexual effectiveness. If you and your partner have a superb sex life, then this will override any possible ways in which you fail to match up to the insidious myth of the 'ideal man'.

The fear: 'I worry that my orgasms are just going to get further and further apart.'

The fact: The sheer lustful ability to come and come and come starts dropping off after the age of seventeen! Once past this sexual peak, both orgasm and ejaculation physically start to take longer, and you may find you need to take longer breaks between orgasms. That's the bad news. The good news is twofold. Firstly, decline is slow; barring ill health, it won't start to affect you until you are approaching retirement, and even then, can be warded off by knowledge, skill and keeping on doing it. Secondly, there are a number of excellent spin-offs to being past the urgency you felt at age seventeen: you can stave off orgasm for longer; you can avoid premature ejaculation; your partner will probably be far more satisfied in the end. But, to make all this work, you need to let go of the panic you may feel if your body is not reacting as it used to do.

The fear: 'Time passing means getting less sexual ... that's the truth.'

The fact: The real truth is that, unless you are in your sixties, any serious drop in sexuality is not down to ageing, but to particular physical or mental blocks that you can almost certainly do something about.

SUPERVIRILITY – THE CHALLENGE

With luck, the previous section has sorted out some of the fears you may have had about your sexuality inevitably fading. But we want to go beyond that. For, as you move beyond the point where sheer physical youth is the driving force behind your sexuality, and get to the age where skill and experience come into their own, new possibilities present themselves. You can last longer, satisfy your partner more fully, and develop your capacity for pleasure.

But only if you face the challenge. So many people have neglected their bodies, limited their mental horizons, become stuck in their relationships and stopped developing their sexual skills. If you want to become Supervirile, you need to look courageously at all these four areas of your life, and face any sexual blocks you may find there.

The challenge of Supervirility is not easy, and that is why, at this early stage, we feel we must point out that not everyone will respond to it. There may be reasons why such a step is the wrong one for you at this present moment.

- You may feel that you are totally satisfied with the sexuality you have now. If so, you don't need this book: keep valuing and loving what you have.

- You may feel some resistance to suggestions on improving your sex life. That's understandable – and this book's approach will not work if you approach it half-heartedly. Put the book away and don't turn to it again, until and unless you want to.

- You may worry that, if you start working on your sexuality, and fail, either you or your partner will start blaming yourselves or each other. This is a logical fear; we want to point out right from the start that, if you don't get the result you want from this programme, that simply means that it isn't the right thing for you at the moment. Don't let anyone, particularly you yourself, start laying blame.

- You may worry that, if you begin improving your sexuality and succeed, this will be too much to handle. How could you, if you wanted to make love all the time? What would be your partner's reaction if you were suddenly totally effective in bed? This is a real worry, and you are right to address it; be reassured that in this book we offer you the skills to let your relationship keep pace with your developing sexuality.

What This Book Does, and How

If you have read this far, you are probably ready to go on to the main body of the book. Before you do so, though, here are a few notes on what it does and does not aim to do and how it is structured.

Supervirility does not:

- offer help if your relationship is non-existent, on the rocks or in crisis. While not expecting you to have an *ideal* relationship, this book does presuppose that you have a relationship to which you are committed, or hope to be committed; it doesn't deal with finding a partner or ironing out serious partnership conflicts;

- offer help with 'primary' sexual blocks. If throughout your life you have never or rarely had any sexual desire, had an erection, been able to penetrate a woman, or been able to ejaculate, then we suggest you see your GP, who may well be able to guide you to the medical or counselling solution you need; or

- offer help with sexual phobia. If you know that you are panicked by the thought of sex, of women, of penetration or of ejaculation, then you need specific counselling tailored to your needs. Appendix A will give you an idea of how to find support.

What does *Supervirility* do? It offers you ways to improve your sexuality through:

- **your body.** Looking at the food you eat; what you drink; any drugs you take; your exercise patterns; your sleep and relaxation patterns; any vulnerability to illness you may have – all with the specific aim of making your body more able to enjoy sex;

- **your mind.** Looking at the way you view sex; the impact of your past on this; the current stresses that are blocking you from responding sexually; the way you could develop your

Introduction

personality to make sexual response more joyful;

- **your relationship.** Examining how your understanding of your partner helps or hinders your ability to make love; the ways in which your relationship may be holding you back from fulfilling your sexual potential; how to overcome any blocks; and

- **your sexual skill.** Exploring your lovemaking; ways of improving technique; your ability to enjoy and prolong sexual fulfilment well beyond the levels you are already enjoying. It offers a step-by-step programme of sexual enhancement through developing technique.

Each of these four parts comprises several chapters. All of these, as well as containing information and explanation, offer you a large number of practical explorations and action plans in order to transfer what you are reading to your everyday life. And thereby hangs a caution.

If you simply read this book, you will learn a great deal. But what you will get from it will be facts, not a super sex life. In order to achieve that, you need to involve yourself in the explorations, series of questions that focus your mind on relevant issues, or sequences of actions that expand your sexual potential. You won't have to do everything we suggest, but where you find a vulnerability, or a lack of knowledge or skill, then you will need to incorporate our suggestions into your life. Some of the practical explorations are rather advanced in format and content; you may need to take a deep breath before daring to do them – but we promise you that they do work.

Equally, in case you need extra support, we suggest at the end of the book that you get further resources from outside – perhaps a relaxation class or a counselling session. Remember that asking for help from outside is not an admission of failure. In the same way, if your television set broke down, you wouldn't think you'd failed if you decided to call in a repairman.

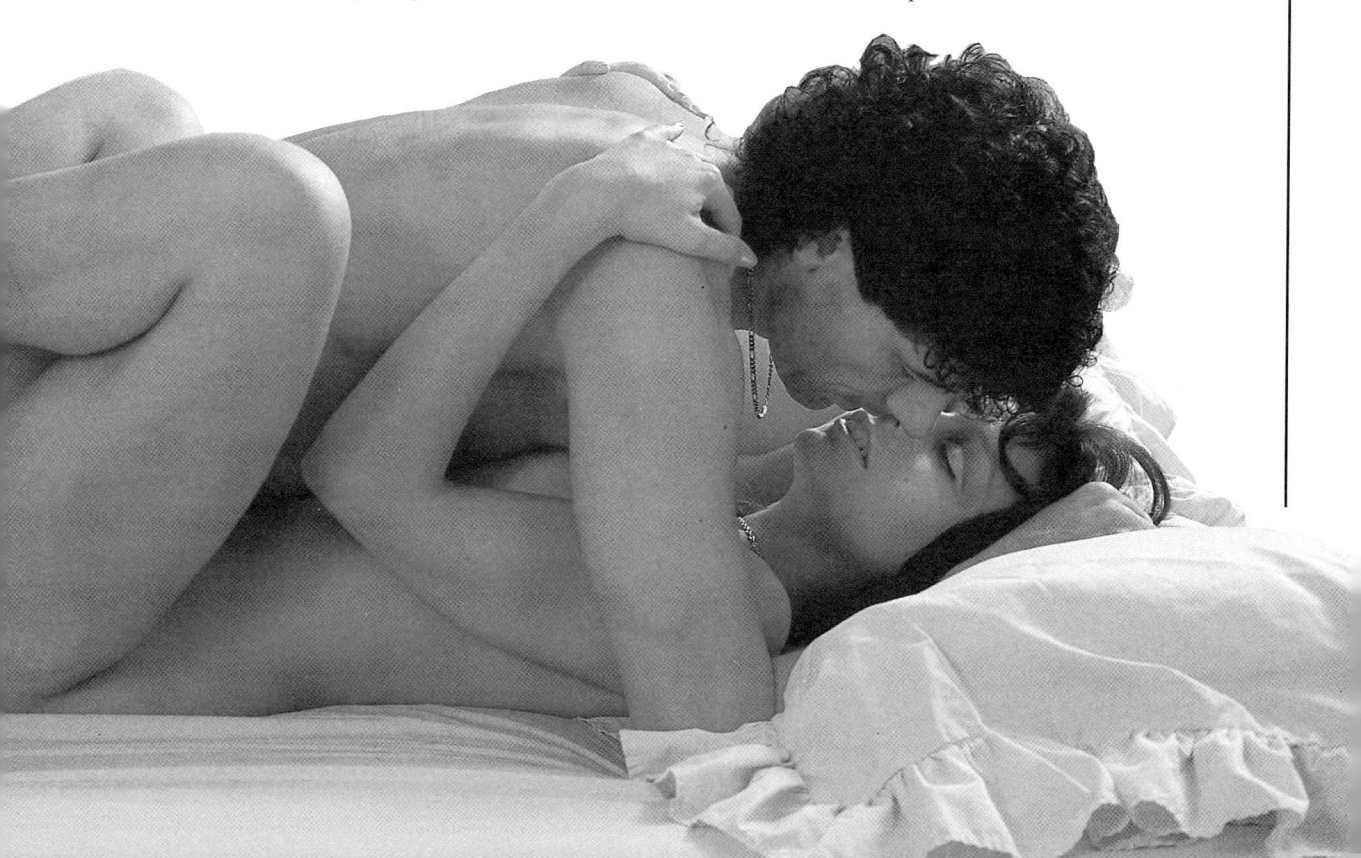

SUPERVIRILITY

Statement	Strongly Agree	Agree	Don't Know	Disagree	Strongly Disagree
1. I know how my body and sexual responses work when my partner and I make love.					
2. I am happy about my weight and size, which is within the healthy range for my build and age.					
3. My diet is well balanced and keeps me fit and healthy.					
4. I drink less than the recommended number of units of alcohol each week.					
5. I don't smoke.					
6. I sleep well.					
7. I wind down easily from work each day.					
8. I take regular exercise.					
9. I feel good about the way I look.					
10. I have no problems with illness or injury... no blood-flow disorders, such as hardening of the arteries (atherosclerosis), no disorders of the nervous system, no hormonal disorders.					
11. I am not currently on any medication.					
12. I got to know about sex in a way that made me feel good about it.					
13. My past sexual relationships have made me increasingly confident and relaxed in bed.					
14. I have not had any severely distressing sexual experiences.					
15. I'm aware when society is trying to feed me pure myths about sexuality.					
16. I find it easy to let go of the stress of everyday life.					
17. I like myself and what I can achieve sexually.					
18. If I can't get an erection, I am happy to let that go and make love some other way.					
19. If I (or my partner) have difficulty coming, I am happy to concentrate on other aspects of love-making.					
20. I am open-minded about sex.					
21. I feel that I know more about my partner as each year goes by.					
22. My partner and I feel our relationship has fully lived up to our expectations.					
23. I feel secure in our relationship and know it is going to last.					
24. My partner and I are able to express our feelings to each other without feeling threatened.					
25. I have no doubt that this is the right relationship for me to be in at present.					
26. In bed, my partner and I are able to support each other when we hit sexual blocks or problems.					
27. I know that my partner is the best option I have for a superb sex life.					
28. Over the years, I have learned more and more about my sexuality and what is possible.					
29. I know how my partner's body works and how it brings her pleasure.					
30. My partner and I know what we want in bed and are able to ask for it.					
31. My partner and I are at ease if one of us initiates sex – or says no to it.					
32. My partner and I often enjoy pre-sexual love play.					
33. Masturbation is a regular part of my sex life, alone and with my partner.					
34. I know many ways to achieve an erection if it doesn't come easily.					
35. I have the technique to achieve penetration even if it doesn't seem easy.					
36. I can choose whether or not to have my orgasm, depending on whether I want to prolong my pleasure or not.					
37. I can let go during my orgasm and really enjoy the pleasure.					
38. After we have made love, my partner and I enjoy spending time together.					
39. I would feel happy to turn to outside help to improve my sexual knowledge and technique.					
40. My partner and I plan to enhance continually our sexuality for as long as we stay together.					

Your Personalized Action Plan

This book isn't meant to be read from cover to cover; it is an action book, which you should read only so far as you need to in order to be able to take action. You will need to know just which elements relevant to your sex life – body, mind, relationship or sexual skill – you need to enhance most.

The exploration on the left takes an overview of elements relevant to gaining and keeping Supervirility. By doing it, you will be guided to the most appropriate parts of the book for you. Read each statement. Beside it, place a mark under the column which most represents your feelings about it: Strongly agree, Agree, Don't know, Disagree, Strongly disagree. Don't linger too long on any one question – your gut reaction is what we want at present.

If you disagree or strongly disagree with any of these statements, they will be areas of vulnerability for you. And, if you answered 'Don't know' to any of them, you are also wise to read the chapter relevant to that point. Your very ignorance may be reducing your sexual potential.

Here are the reasons why each question is vital, along with the chapters of the book that cover the relevant issues.

1. Finding out how your sexuality works will enhance your experience, not spoil it. Chapter 1.

2. Too much weight stresses your whole system, so will cut down your capacity for strenuous and effective sex. Chapter 2.

3. Unless you are eating the right food, your body can't respond sexually. Chapter 2.

4. Drinking more than a small amount of alcohol may mean that you can't get an erection. Chapter 2.

5. Smoking has a number of horrific effects on your sex life. Chapter 2.

6. Lack of sleep can undermine your sexuality very quickly. Chapter 2.

7. If you are overworked and cannot wind down then your entire body may be saying no to sex. Chapter 2.

8. Exercise is vital to keep your body systems working, help you move freely during sex and make you look good. Chapter 2.

9. Feeling bad about your body and the way you use it undermines your sexual performance. Chapters 3 and 9.

10. Some illnesses, injuries or operations, blood-flow disorders, nervous system disorders and decreased production of male hormones can cause sexual difficulty. Chapter 4.

11. Some medications affect your sexuality. Chapter 4.

12. Exactly how we first learn about sex can be crucial to how much pleasure we can get from it later on. Chapter 6.

13. Past relationships can teach us unhelpful lessons about sexuality. Chapter 6.

14. A sexual trauma can affect our sexuality for life. Chapter 6.

15. Society has a large number of myths about sex which stop us fulfilling our sexual potential. Chapter 7.

16. Stress can stop us feeling desire or being able to make love. Chapter 8.

17. Our self-esteem comes through clearly in bed, and will affect our love-making. Chapter 9.

18. The starting point for most erectile dysfunction is often not the body's failure to get it up, but our mental worry about that. Chapter 9.

19. Being able to relax and enjoy love-making without worry about orgasm or ejaculation is crucial to good sex. Chapter 9.

20. Accepting all aspects of love-making, body intimacy and innovations will keep our sex life constantly developing. Chapter 9.

21. Updated knowledge of your partner, her past and present, is essential if you are to have a truly intimate relationship. Chapter 10.

22. Disillusionment is one of the key factors that can undermine desire and sexual potential in a relationship. Chapter 11.

23. Fear and anxiety within a partnership is the other main factor that can prevent love-making from being fulfilling. Chapter 11.

24. An ability constantly to express feelings is a way to ensure that desire does not die. Chapter 12.

25. Solid sexual partnerships are founded on a desire to stay together. Chapter 12.

26. Acceptance of sexual blocks or inhibitions, plus commitment to overcome them, is part of all good sexual partnerships. Chapter 12.

27. You need to be aware of the alternatives for sexual fulfilment – in order to know that you are still committed to your partner. Chapter 13.

28. As time passes, you need to update your knowledge and sexual technique in order to keep interest alive. Chapter 14.

29. Knowing just how your partner likes to be aroused is crucial to success in bed. Chapter 14.

30. A mutual ability to ask, receive and give in bed enables you to get exactly what you want. Chapter 15.

31. For either of you to be able to initiate sex – or say no to it – gives you an equality in bed that is vital. Chapter 15.

32. The lead-up to sex is an essential part of sex itself. Chapters 15 and 16.

33. Masturbation helps you to increase your pleasure potential – and continually helps your partner learn what pleases you. Chapter 17.

34. Knowing how to get an erection when it seems difficult is useful in love-making. Chapter 18.

35. Achieving penetration when that seems tricky is an essential skill. Chapter 20.

36. Being able to continue love-making without orgasm may mean that you can make love more often and for longer. Chapter 21.

37. Enjoying orgasm fully means that you are able to lose yourself in the sensations of sex. Chapter 21.

38. The period after sex is crucial to building love in preparation for next time. Chapter 21.

39. Looking outside for support when you hit blocks means that you increase your chance of sexual success. Appendices A and B.

40. Planning an even more wonderful sex life together than you already have, and being committed to working towards that, will guarantee you Supervirility. Chapter 21.

Now you have pinpointed what you need to know and to do, read on. Make your way through the book, taking from it what you need. If at any time you feel you are losing your way, repeat this questionnaire, checking just where you are in your journey towards Supervirility, and finding out exactly what you need to do next, in order to get there.

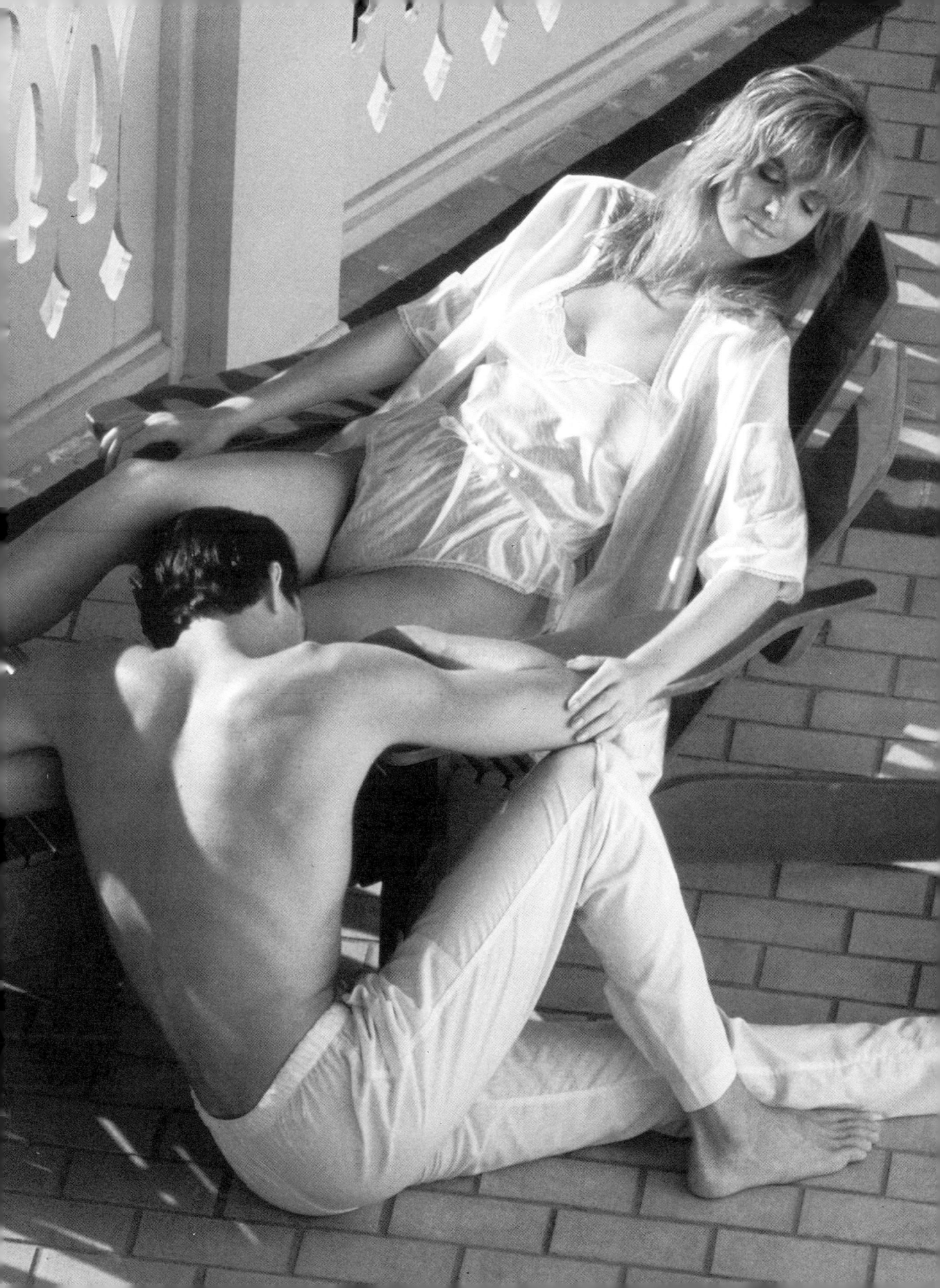

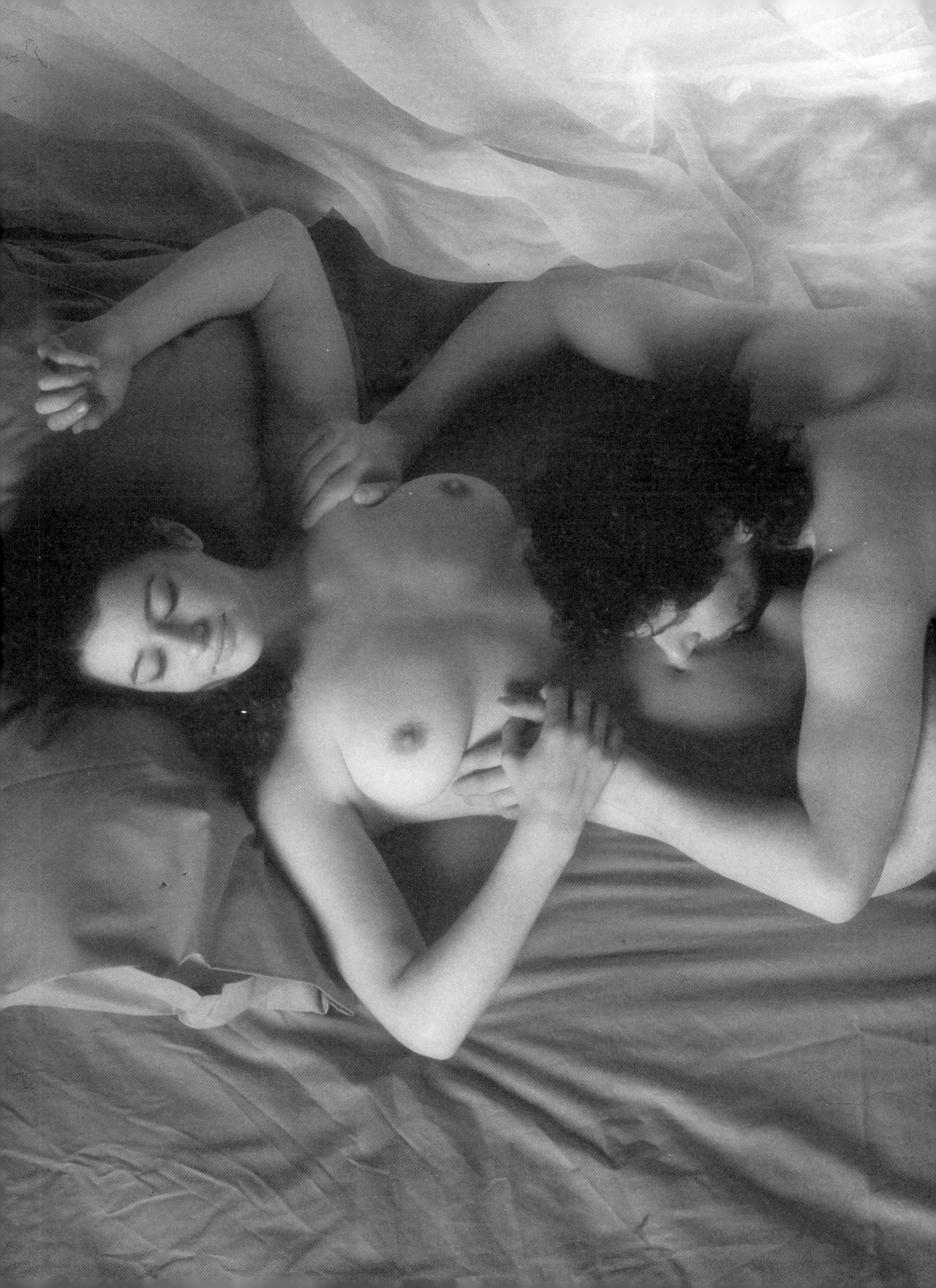

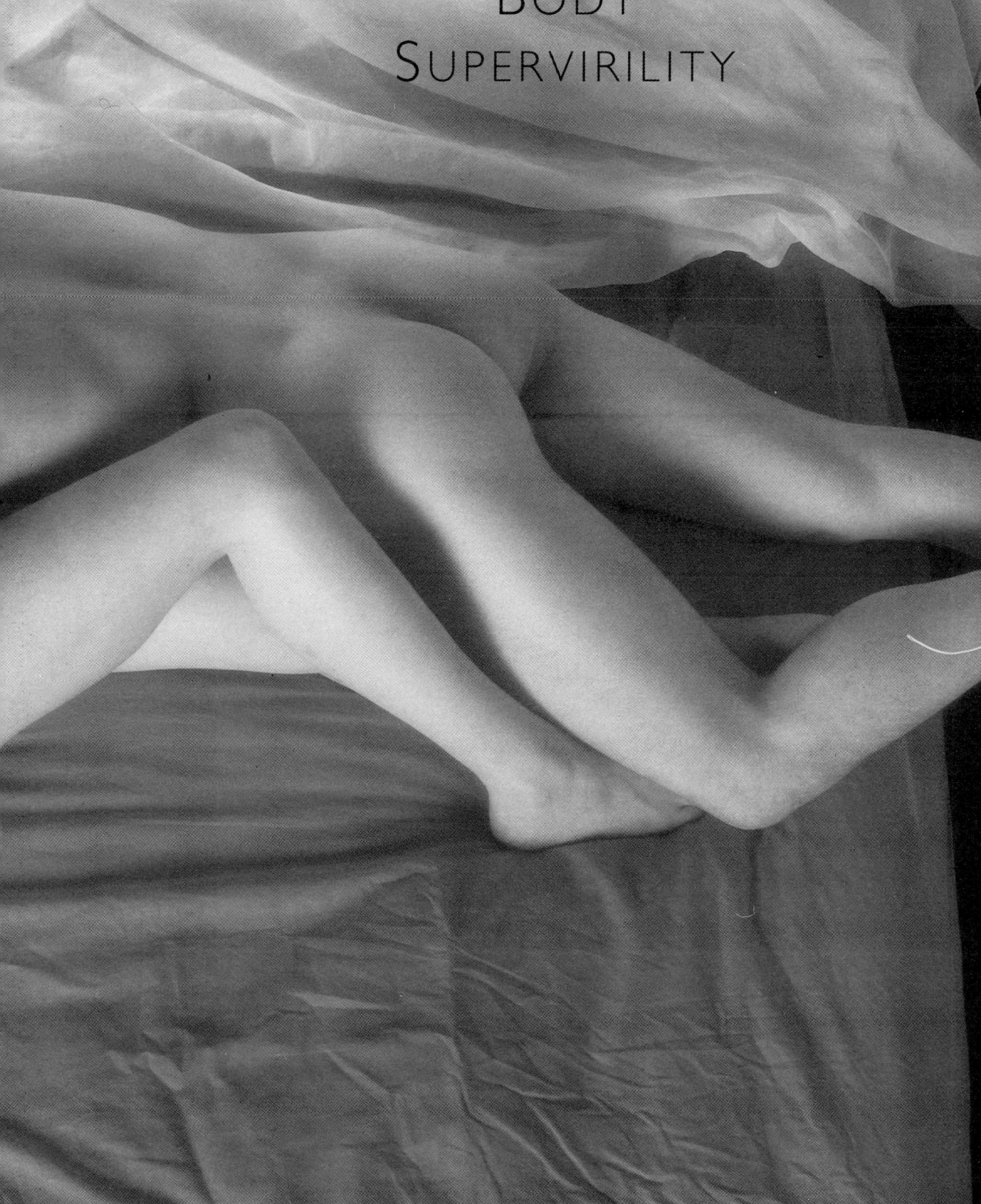

PART I
BODY
SUPERVIRILITY

SUPERVIRILITY

Your Body, Your Sexuality

In order to be Supervirile, our bodies have to work well. We want them to be physically attractive to us and to our partner, to react when we want them to, and to be healthy so that no illness gets in the way of sex. This section, on body Supervirility, outlines the ways in which you can ensure that your body is a functioning sexual tool – and that any problems you have with it are resolved before they affect your sex life.

This first chapter is a quick tour of the male body, how it works and what can go wrong with its sexual functioning. This will give you the knowledge you need to start making informed decisions about your fitness and health. To add practical experience to this knowledge, we suggest that you take a very direct part in this particular tour. We suggest that you conduct it with and upon your own body.

THE GUIDED TOUR

The best way to begin is to stand in front of a full-length mirror. Perhaps you can do this after a bath, when you are naked anyway; make sure you aren't disturbed by your partner or family, so you can concentrate fully on the experience. You'll need to take about half an hour, reading and looking as you go, to make this tour.

First, take a general look. Relax; you're not alone in disliking large areas of your body, and feeling that they could be different. Every man has lurked in and out of changing rooms hoping that no one will notice him! The truth is that only a very small proportion of men look like the models in the magazines or in the movies, and those models are only paid large amounts of money because they are so unusual. Most men are of average height, weight and attractiveness. And they don't look like film stars.

Next, start getting to grips with how your body works.

Look closely at **the way you are built,** the way you stand, the way the muscles hang on your body. Try moving a hand, an arm, a leg, and realizing that it is this combination of muscles, nerves, blood and bone that enables you to make love. Notice the fine details of your body, such as hair, its texture and colour; your eyes and how they are set in their sockets; the shape of your nose, ears and mouth; your fingers – and toenails. Notice any features of your body that mark you out, any birthmarks, scars or special features.

Your **senses** are the route by which erotic stimuli first reach you. Try closing your eyes or blocking your ears to experience what it is like to be without these senses. When you open your eyes, notice that they register not only shape and size, but also tiny gradations of colour, pattern and position. When you unblock your ears, realize that they register not only noise in the room, but the finest differences of pitch, tone and volume. And although what you see or hear may be the first things you are aware of, in fact it is smell which most immediately arouses you. The scent or taste of your partner will affect you many times more quickly than will the sight or sound of her. The point in becoming aware of all this is to begin to develop the channels of your senses, which through their five routes bring you all the information you get during love-making. Later, you can start to train your senses to respond at a higher level, to achieve greater and more sensuous sexuality.

Covering the entire body is the **skin,** our most vital erogenous zone. Under the surface of the skin are nerves, which carry erotic sensation. Try touching your own skin, charting where it is most sensitive, and where least. The neck, mouth, insides of thighs, buttocks, ear lobes, breasts, the insides of your arms, the lips, mouth and tongue are all likely to be sensitive – and you will also have erogenous zones that are individual to you. As you touch, be aware of the particular sensations that you feel, the way they travel to your genitals from the spot you are touching. Beyond your awareness, they also carry messages to the brain, telling your entire system that something is happening.

Next, think about the **blood system** that serves your body; you can probably see its tiny network of veins under the skin if you look on the inside of your wrist. In general terms, arteries and veins carry oxygen from lungs to brain, and then round to all parts of your body, including the nervous system, muscles and main organs. Blood supplies energy to them all and thus allows them to sense, feel and move. In particular, blood flow is essential to your genitals – for it is blood that fills your penis each time you have an erection.

The brain has been called the most important sexual organ. The limbic system, located at the back rim of the brain, is currently reckoned to be the spot where erotic impulses are received when the five senses are stimulated. This spot links with other parts of the brain, making key connections that send messages down the spinal cord and along the nerves to the genitals. As the penis is stimulated, messages are sent back to the brain confirming that you are feeling pleasure. But, equally, if something somewhere occurs to convince your brain that sex is not a good idea, messages are sent to inhibit your response. Nerve reaction fades, as does your experience of desire.

At the same time, **hormones** – chemical substances produced in various glands – move round the body arousing it to action. Although scientists are unclear about exactly what part it plays, the male hormone testosterone seems to be the 'libido' chemical that most creates sexual arousal. It is clear that any illness causing an imbalance of testosterone can lead to a diminishing of desire and make it difficult for you to get an erection. What is not so clear is how you can ensure a good supply of testosterone in your body.

THE PRIVATE PARTS

Now pay attention to your more erogenous zones.

First, look at your **nipples**. Perhaps, for you, these are not sensitive – but for many men they are an essential area of arousal. Try touching them lightly, and bearing them in mind for further attention next time you make love.

Then look down at your **penis.** Whether limp or erect, you probably think it seems smaller than you would want. But here lies a great sexual secret.

Most men feel that their penis is smaller than they would like. Many of them believe that their erect penis is smaller than other men's... But... Most erect penises are exactly the same size!

If you already knew this, and are truly at ease with your penis size, accept our congratulations. You are rare. The majority of men have been conned by fate and the media into believing that they are lacking in some way.

If you look down at yourself again, and then look across at yourself in the mirror, you will see one very good reason why most men fall for the con. A penis seen from above looks a lot smaller than one seen from directly in front. In other words, if you look across at other men's penises in the changing room and then look down at your own, you will think that yours is smaller.

Of course, if you look up at a man's penis shown in a dirty movie, where camera angles collude to make the whole thing seem three inches bigger than it really is, you will feel even worse. The huge penis is almost always a figment of someone's imagination.

Worries aside, you may now want to look at your private parts more closely. You may think that, after all these years of holding yourself several times a day, you know well enough what you are like. In fact, you probably don't know yourself as well as you think you do. Have a closer look as you ask yourself these questions.

How would you describe your penis when non-erect?

How dark a colour is it, what shape and size?

How does the skin hang over the tip if you are uncircumcised, or pull back from it if you are circumcised?

What shape is the glans of the penis – flat, angular, curved in exactly what way – and how does the colour change on each part of the glans? Look and touch too the frenulum, the tiny band of ultra-sensitive skin that connects the under-surface of the glans to the foreskin.

Use your fingers gently to move the skin of the penis back and forth.

Inside, there are two tubes of tissue beneath the skin, waiting to fill up with blood when you are erect, while a third carries the urethra or urinary passage which not only brings your urine from your bladder, but also brings the semen when the time comes. All these tubes continue into your body, into the pelvic area to connect with organs, muscles and blood vessels.

Carry on exploring your **scrotum**. Inside this sac of skin are the testicles, the glands which produce the sperm that are carried in your ejaculate. Again, you may want to explore, feeling just how large your testicles are – most are similar in size to a large grape – and just what shape. Look in the mirror at the colour of the skin that covers them, and how they can have a disconcerting habit of moving position according to how aroused (or how warm or cold) you are.

Inside your testicles, a complex battery of glands and tubes link the testes and the penis. The prostate gland, situated at the back of the body above your anus, produces the fluid that carries the sperm. The seminal vesicles also secrete a thick fluid that helps the sperm survive. From both these, and from the Cowper's glands which lie just below the prostate, comes fluid which makes up your ejaculate.

WHEN YOU GET AROUSED

Now think about how your body responds during successful lovemaking. We have already said that when **desire** strikes, and you first see something that turns you on, your brain and hormonal system work in tandem to send messages round your body.

If all goes well, the messages from the brain and the hormones create **arousal**. Energized by oxygen pulled in by your lungs, blood rushes into the penis, through arteries that widen for the process and through penile tissues that expand. Your penis becomes filled with blood – and, because at the same time the veins that normally drain blood from the penis become compressed, the penis remains full of that blood, rising to **erection**.

Simultaneously, other changes are occurring all over your body. Your pulse rate and breathing may rise, your nostrils may flare, your nipples may become erect, your muscles tense, pupils enlarge and your testes rise closer to your body.

As your **excitement** mounts, your penis swells until it is fully erect. Its tip may become darker, your testicles swell even more, and a few drops of lubricating fluid may ooze from the head of your penis, preparing it for penetration. Increasingly, your breath and heart rate will rise and, beyond your conscious awareness, your blood pressure is mounting, your nervous system is rising to the challenge.

Before orgasm, there is what is known as the **plateau phase**. Here, arousal is at the highest point it can reach; your body hovers in a state of total excitement, with all pleasure systems at full pitch, waiting only for the final stimulation before tipping over into orgasm.

Then, it happens. There is a two-part process, though sometimes the two parts seem to occur together. First, **orgasm** feels inevitable; you pass the point of no return and all your genital muscles contract in one huge movement. Then, the prostate glands and the seminal vesicles expel their fluid; the contractions of orgasm, one every 0.8 seconds, cause this semen to rush through the urethra to be ejaculated out of the tip of the penis – up to 600 million sperm in one go!

Afterwards, all returns to normal. The brain stops sending arousal messages, and the hormones cease flooding your system. Your nervous system returns to its former state, as do your muscles; heart rate, breathing and blood pressure go back to normal. In your penis, arteries dilate and veins expand to let the blood flow out, the direct opposite of the process which enabled erection. Your penis goes soft, the scrotum descends, and you enter the **relaxation** or refractory period (the word refractory means 'incapable of stimulation'). You can't become erect again for a while, even if you want to; however energetic you feel, your whole system – brain, hormones, nervous system, heart, blood flow – all need a rest.

WHEN BLOCKS ARISE

What we have just described is the usual pattern of arousal. In fact, as with all activities in life, men vary in their reactions and also vary according to the time, the place, the mood and, very importantly, according to the partner they are with. Sometimes all the positive elements occur together, and love-making is perfect.

More often, for everyone except the models in the dirty movies, it doesn't happen like this. In fact, sex is not wonderful all the time for everyone but you. In *The Kinsey New Report on Sex,* forty-nine per cent of men said that they had suffered sexual dissatisfaction at some time in their life. And these are just the ones who admitted it.

For the fact is that, whether through directly physical causes, or because physical response is affected by mental state, often enough sexual response can fall short of what is required. Perhaps you don't feel as desirous as you would like, gain an erection as easily as you'd wish, feel as much pleasure in love-making as you could, or know that your partner is not as fulfilled as possible. To iron out any possible blocks in your sex life, you need to understand exactly what is happening physically when, for some reason, you fail to get all you want from love-making.

First, you need to consider what happens as you go through different stages in life. At seventeen, all our body systems are at peak performance; brain, muscles, nerves, blood flow and hormones all combining to urge us on to sex, Nature's way of hinting that now is the best time for us to be making babies. No wonder we spend a great deal of our time in a permanent state of arousal!

In the normal course, parts of the body do have some built-in obsolescence. Our senses may become less acute, as we become more short-sighted or lose our peak hearing. Our body may begin to lose its hair, particularly on our heads. Skin gradually loses its elasticity and becomes drier or calloused with work. Because of the stresses and strains of life, and the negative effects of some of the things we eat and drink, we can end up with clogged arteries, or organs that are more vulnerable than they were. With less energy as we age, we can take less exercise, and so our muscles lose their tone and we gain weight. Our brain remains active, but slowly our nervous system begins to fall from peak performance; our hormones may level off and become less effective.

It sounds horrific, but it is in fact just a red herring. We have outlined the effects of ageing so that we can, immediately, point

Your Body, Your Sexuality

out that it is nonsense to think that ageing means we cannot have sex. This is what Helen Singer-Kaplan, the sex therapist who brought the whole issue of fading desire to public attention in the early 1980s, calls 'one of the great fallacies of our culture'. She points out that the natural ageing changes we've just described are subtle; they may stop us running a marathon (though some men in their seventies do just that) but, barring illness, they may not have any real impact on our sex lives until we are well into our sixties. Even then, with physical care, due warning and the right mental outlook, negative sexual side-effects can be staved off for many years – while the positive effects of ageing can be a positive enhancement to our ability in bed. It is how we treat our bodies, our minds and our partners, not the natural passing of time, that most dictates the quality of our sex life. So let us lay the myth of ageing aside for good, and concentrate on what we can do here and now to promote Super-virility.

What might you be doing physically to prevent your body from attaining peak sexual condition? Let us examine possible sexual blocks and consider what their physical roots may be.

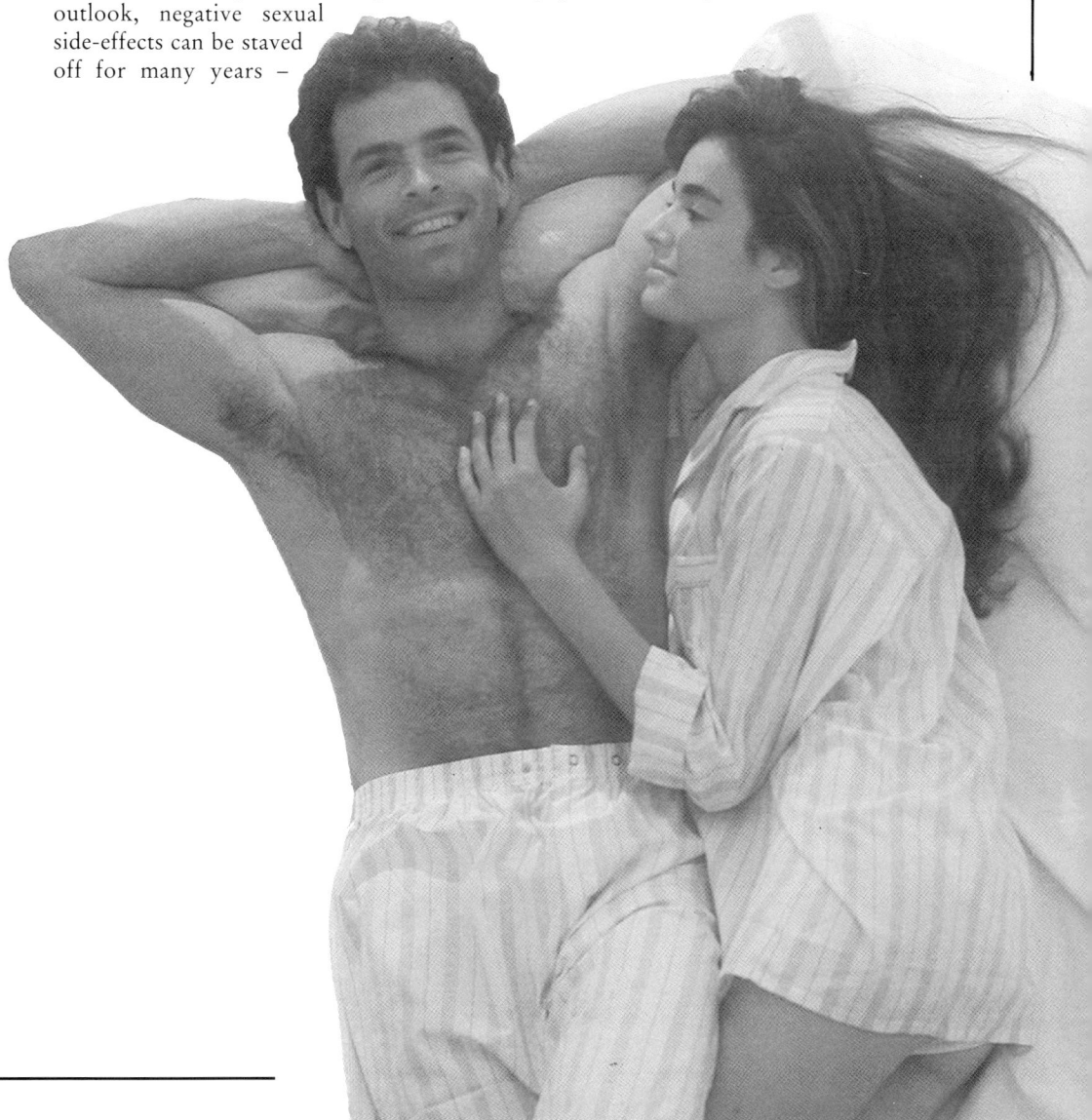

- If **desire** is lacking, then somewhere your initial physical response to erotic stimuli has been dulled. Perhaps you are putting yourself under strain, perhaps illness is affecting your reactions, perhaps you are not nourishing your body sufficiently. Whatever the cause, the areas affected will involve your whole body system. Perhaps you are unable to feel desire through the five channels of the senses. Perhaps your hormones are failing to carry the relevant chemical messages around your body. Perhaps your nervous system, from brain through spinal cord to every part of you, is failing to respond. Perhaps your brain itself is receiving contradictory messages, suggesting desire but then inhibiting it at the same time – through the physical messages of pain in any part of your body, or through the chemicals produced by stress or anxiety. This can happen through directly physical means, although, as we explain later in the book, more often it is through the thoughts we have about ourselves and our sexual relationships.

- If desire is there, but **erection** does not follow or cannot be sustained, then there may be many possible reasons for it. Physically, three elements of your system may be particularly affected. There may be an imbalance in your hormones, which are failing to indicate that erection is needed. It may be that some blockage in your blood supply is stopping the blood necessary for erection from entering your penis – or making it too easy for the blood to leave your penis, thus leading to the same end result. It may be that the particular part of your nervous system responsible for genital arousal is in some way failing to respond. All these responses may be triggered biologically or psychologically, by some blockage in the body or in your mental approach.

- In the **excitement** and **plateau phase** of love-making, when heartbeat, blood pressure and breathing rate are high, and when movement may vary from slow and gentle through to violently energetic, then your whole body determines whether you are able to fulfil your potential. What holds you back here is your capacity to breathe, to move, to endure high levels of heart and lung activity.

- Not being able to enjoy completely the pleasures of the plateau phase is more often an issue for younger men than for older. What happens in biological terms is that the mechanisms of emission and expulsion kick in sooner than you want them to: the pelvic area responding, the prostate gland and seminal vesicles moving into action, and the whole orgasmic cycle overwhelming all your good intentions. The result is **premature ejaculation**. Again, this can all be affected either physically or psychologically.

- Conversely, delay in orgasm will be due to the mechanisms of emission and expulsion kicking in much later than you want them to. This is, not surprisingly, called **delayed ejaculation**, and could be due to some kind of disorder of the nerves in your pelvic region, which in turn may be due to both physical and psychological factors of various kinds. Not being able to come at all is a rare condition, but as you get older, extended periods of love-making without reaching orgasm get more likely. As we will be discussing later in the book, once placed in their proper context, these are actually good news.

- The fullness and satisfaction of orgasm may vary from time to time, depending on how well your whole body is working on each occasion. And although this is unlikely to affect the satisfaction of your orgasm, the strength and amount of your **ejaculation** may also vary – the spurt being more or less powerful, and the volume greater or lesser. Barring injury, however, it will always contain sperm.

- The sense of release and pleasure after love-making is often wonderful. What may be less than ideal is the **relaxation time**, the pause before it can all begin again – and here we pedal back to the initial phase of the sexual cycle. How long does it take before you are able to feel desire again, before your brain, hormones, blood flow and nervous system are ready to respond? Certainly, if for some reason any of these elements of your body system are not in peak condition then it will take longer for them to react. This is particularly true after ejaculation, which seems to deplete the body not only of semen, but also of the energy and motivation to move into the desire phase once more.

In this final part of the chapter we have looked at the potential areas of your sexuality which may need enhancement – in the rest of this section you will be looking at possible physical ways of achieving this enhancement, and in other sections of the book you will be looking at possible ways of enhancement that involve your mind, relationship and sexual skill. However, before you move on to learning in detail how to maximize your potential, take a moment to check the elements of your sexual response that you already, instinctively, feel need some enhancement – so that, as you read on, you will know what needs particular attention:

- your level of physical desire – the amount or the frequency of desire to make love;

- your levels of excitement and erection – whether erection comes as easily, stays as firm or lasts as long as you would wish;

- your ability to hold off from coming for as long as you want to, particularly when you are in the plateau phase of high arousal;

- your ability to come quickly and easily enough; and

- the length of time it takes before you are ready for love-making again.

Notice that we specify no times or levels of quality or quantity in asking these questions. For there are no meaningful standards in sexuality; if you and your partner are happy with your love-making, however long or short the time it takes, however high or low your level of excitement, then that is right for you. If you are not happy, whatever you are doing in bed, then it is possible to change.

SUPERVIRILITY

BUILDING YOUR BODY

2

For true Supervirility, you need a body that will rise to the challenge. So it is vital to make sure that everything you eat, drink or inhale adds positively to your Supervirility – and that your body is given enough chance to both recuperate and to stretch to its limits.

By now, you may well be mentally crawling under the nearest stone, convinced that in this chapter we will be telling you to eat only lettuce leaves, drink only water, and jog round the block five times a day.

Certainly, the guidelines we suggest are sensible, but we hope they are also enjoyable in the short term as well as in the long term. And, if there is one overriding rule, it is this: take any changes slowly and don't try to do everything at once. For Supervirility is about enjoying life to the full, out of bed as well as in it. And if by following our guidelines you become a self-denying grouch, you will not enjoy sex and neither will your partner.

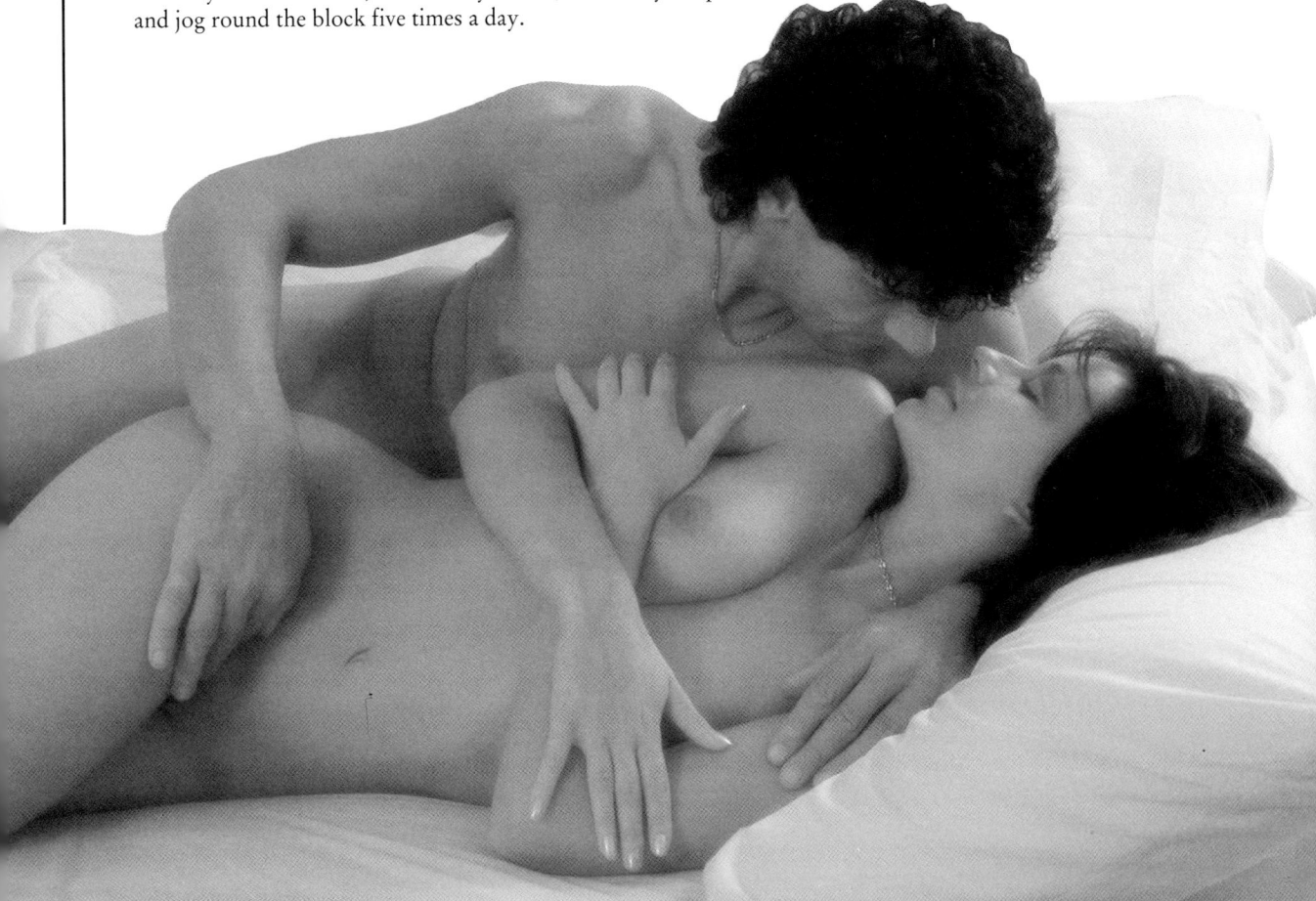

Food For Love

Your first step has to be assessing your diet for its Supervirility effect. Take a look in your fridge and your larder, and answer the following questions:

- How much frozen, tinned, processed or cook-chill food is there, versus fresh, unprocessed or organically grown food? The more processed a food is, the less nutritional value it is likely to have – making your physical appearance less attractive and draining the energy you need for sex.

- How much low-fibre food is there (white bread and pasta, refined breakfast cereal, products made with white flour) versus high-fibre wholemeal bread, rice, breakfast cereal, pasta, beans and pulses, and whole vegetables? High-fibre foods help your digestion, stave off bowel cancers, keep you trim and so flexible and energetic in bed.

- How much high-fat food such as cream, milk, butter, oil and fried food is there, versus low-fat food (low-fat spreads and oils, skimmed milk, yoghurt, polyunsaturated fats such as those found in vegetable oils, olive oil and avocado pears)? Fatty foods or foods fried in fat pile on the weight, as well as increasing the risk of heart disease, leaving you possibly unable to gain an erection.

- How much sugary food is there – sweets, biscuits, cakes, ice cream, sweetened drinks, glucose or fructose drinks? As well as adding weight sugar ruins your teeth – and contains no nutrients at all.

Next, look at whether any of these foods are creating a bad reaction in you. In these days of chemically produced food, a single allergic reaction can sap your energy and turn off sexuality as completely as turning off a tap. If you know that every time you eat or drink something, you feel odd or ill afterwards, try cutting out that substance for a week. You may miss it at first, but after a while, you won't. Then reintroduce just a small helping into your diet, and see what the reaction is; if it is bad enough, you simply won't be tempted to eat that food again.

Make sure too that you are eating at the right time of day for you. Social rules specify breakfast, lunch, tea, dinner or supper, a big meal at night and occasional snacks. But people are different and you need to discover what suits you. We personally find that eating heavily makes us drowsy, so we have a light meal if we know we are going to make love!

Thirdly, eat only as much as will maintain your ideal weight. You don't need us to tell you that an overweight body is less sexy to look at and less erotic to hold. Don't cut down radically on what you eat – because then your body thinks it's starving and desperately clings on to the food you offer, turning it into fat! Instead, replace anything you eat that isn't highly nutritious with high-nutrient foods. This will give you more energy to burn off the food you are eating. Next, replace high-fat or high-sugar foods with low-fat or low-sugar alternatives, thereby reducing calories painlessly. Learn to tell when you are actually full. Stop eating. The bottom line is that a human stomach is roughly the size of a closed fist, and if you have more food than this on your plate, you are eating more than your body can handle immediately. Guess what happens to the overflow... straight on to the waistline!

Sexual supplements

Through the food you eat, you should be getting sufficient vitamins and minerals. Until you feel you are up to peak health and sexuality, however, begin by taking a good daily general vitamin and mineral supplement. After that, eat sensibly, supplementing when you feel you are under stress, bearing in mind that some vitamins are particularly vital for feeding the Supervirility parts of your body.

- The B vitamins (found in wholegrain products, nuts, seeds, egg yolk, oily fish, bananas and avocados) help your brain and nervous system – both essential to get arousal going.

- Vitamin C (in fresh fruit, green vegetables and potatoes) helps keep your hormone levels stable, and is particularly vital if you smoke or are prone to infection.

- Vitamin E (in nuts, seeds, avocado oils and fish oils) promotes the elasticity of skin and has a reputation for staving off the effects of ageing. It helps keep your blood vessel walls in good shape and so keeps penile blood-flow disorders at bay; some studies claim that a deficiency of Vitamin E causes impotence.

- Zinc is a trace mineral found in the prostate gland and in sperm. Zinc deficiency is associated with sexual disorders and prostate disease, and, by logical reversal, it has been suggested that a sufficient quantity of zinc in your body makes you virile. But don't overdo it; a zinc overdose can cause bad reactions. Instead, eat a diet rich in whole grains, fresh peas, carrots and milk – and remember the Eastern European saying 'seeds for the seed'. You may, of course, want to make absolutely sure you have no deficiency by treating yourself to that famous virility food, zinc-rich oysters!

Stimulating stimulants

While a small amount of the stimulants found in everyday drinks such as coffee, tea and cocoa can seem to give you more energy and stamina for erotic night-time activities, mounting research proves that regular drinking stresses your nervous system – the vital network for all aspects of sexuality. You may feel edgy and irritable, not the best basis for love-making; you may be easily distracted, unable to lose yourself in erotic sensation.

We differ on this. Ian drinks instant coffee regularly, would hate to give it up and finds himself feeling bad only if he has more than several cups a day. Sue stopped drinking coffee and tea over twenty years ago and finds that even one cup sends her berserk! Our advice is to moderate your intake; try replacing coffee and tea with milky drinks or herb teas at least part of the time, maybe cutting down from six cups a day to two. If, when you go back to the stimulants, your body shrieks, then you may have to choose between them and your sexuality!

Drink to me only...

Sexually, alcohol is a double-edged sword. It tastes and smells nice, and the first drink at any rate makes you feel good. The all-over body warmth and flushing, the sensation of thinking more effectively and feeling more deeply is incredibly seductive – if drinking is occasional.

Regular drinking is something very different. Alcohol goes to all the private parts that other substances don't reach, and renders them vulnerable. In the short term, your penis becomes less sensitive, and may decide not to perform: twelve hours after six pints of average-strength beer, sex hormone levels may still be low enough to stop you feeling desire at all. Long-term effects can be even worse: alcohol slows or eliminates ejaculation, reduces your sperm count, and increases the amount of the female hormone oestrogen in your body. All the above is relevant, incidentally, even if you personally feel no ill-effects or hangovers.

After all this you may, as we ourselves did, be nervously wondering whether to give up alcohol altogether. The answer is that, unless you have a serious drink problem, there is no need to give up, but you may want to think about cutting down.

The aim is to follow these guidelines:

- drink no more than twenty-one units a week (fourteen for women). One unit is a glass of wine or spirits, a half-pint of ordinary beer or a quarter pint of extra-strength beer;

- drink day-on, day-off to give your nervous system and hormones a chance to recover; and

- if you binge, keep off alcohol for several days afterwards – binges may tip your system over into lifelong vulnerability.

Light my fire – or not

Smoking may seem like a good idea when you start. By the time you've been smoking for years, it seems to help you relax, give you something to do with your hands, even keep the weight off.

But what does it do to your sex life? It is ironic that the icon of post-coital bliss used to be to light up a cigarette. The fact is that the blissful couple smoking together in the 1950s cinema romance are probably by now physically incapable of more than a goodnight kiss! Tobacco smoke, a recent Health Education Authority (HEA) leaflet tells us, contains 4000 chemicals. It ruins your breathing, thereby depriving you of strength and stamina. It interferes with your sensory acuity so that your senses cannot stimulate you to desire. It depresses your hormone levels, lowers your sperm count – and to add insult to injury, decreases the amount of blood flowing into your penis, so ultimately, your erection will suffer. The aim, it has to be said, must be to stop smoking; alternatively, you need to accept that you will always have a sex life that is below par.

What of drugs?

Hard drugs like heroin or cocaine will ultimately screw up your system so much that sex will be a total irrelevance to you, and in our opinion only fools get hooked into that. We presume that if you are reading this you are not a fool, so will confine ourselves to discussing soft drugs.

On the one hand, there is extensive expert research showing that most of the social drugs used currently depress sensual response, lowering sex drive and arousal by affecting the nervous system and hormone production. Conversely, it is arguable – and many medical and legal experts have argued this – that most soft drugs are actually no more harmful to you than alcohol is. Equally, the subjective experience may well be that soft drugs make sex a more sensual, sensitive experience. We would suggest that just as one bottle of wine is occasionally a nice way to enhance love-making – but not something to rely on – occasional use of social stimulants is another way to enhance sex. If your performance starts to suffer, you start to rely on them for pleasure, or if your partner reacts negatively, then stop at once.

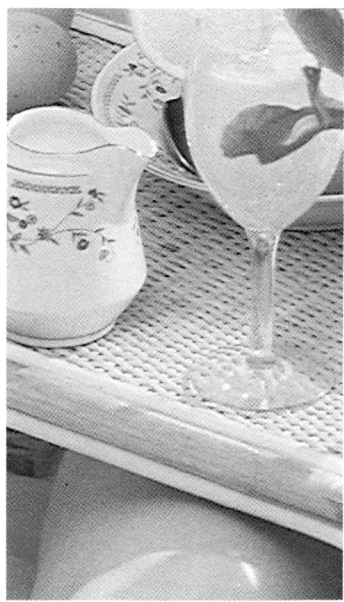

Sleeping Soundly

Sleep is a built-in survival system, allowing all parts of the body to renew themselves and get ready for the day. It is no coincidence that, when you wake in the morning, you often have an erection: your hormone levels are highest then, your nerves and organs are rested and ready to go.

To ensure peak virility, make sure you get enough quality sleep for your needs. To really benefit, you need to relax sufficiently to drop to the deepest levels of sleep, where brain waves move to a different pattern; this is only possible if you are comfortable and secure. So check. Is the bed wide enough, soft or hard enough, are the bedclothes the right weight, can you stretch and move during sleep to allow real relaxation? Are you timing your sleep correctly; if you are an 'early-morning' person, the hours between ten and six are probably best for you while a 'night person' may need to sleep between midnight and eight o'clock for best results.

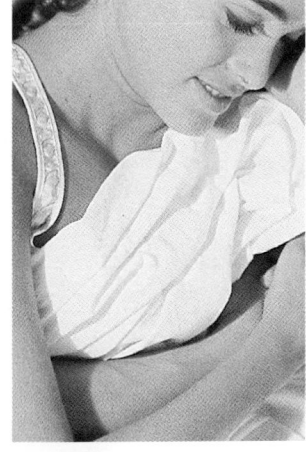

Relaxing for Pleasure

Every day, particularly if you are working at peak performance, challenges will stress your body. The hormone adrenaline will flood your system, and the after-effect will hit all the systems involved in sexuality: your shallow breath will fail to energize your blood; your overstretched nerves will become less able to respond.

Unless by regular relaxation you give your body a chance to recover, its response when asked to perform at the end of the day will be to withdraw from the fray. Alternatively, it may leap into sex with a 'For heaven's sake, let's get it over with' approach, turning the whole thing into yet another stressful experience that lacks enjoyment.

How can you learn to relax? First, take regular, brief breaks. Become aware of your own physical tension (usual trouble spots are tummy, back, neck) when at work, as your shoulders rise tensely or your voice begins to get harsh and stressed. Whenever this happens, there are many things you can do which won't be noticed even in the most formal work meeting. Adjust your posture to a more relaxed one by shifting in your chair or raising and lowering your shoulders. Stretch slightly, legs under the table, arms down by your sides. Breathe deeply and calmly three times. Yawn, or pretend to yawn.

Also, take more lengthy relaxation each day. Five minutes is enough, at your desk, in your car after a long drive, or on a park bench during the lunch hour. Get comfortable, then tense up each part of your body in turn, breathe out and then relax that part. Chart the difference between tense and relaxed, and so get more effect. To come back to the real world without tensing up again, stretch, yawn and look up to the sky or ceiling while you count slowly backwards from ten.

At the end of the day, for full relaxation, take a transition period to allow yourself to wind down at home. Avoid the classic before-dinner drink, which increases reliance on alcohol. Instead, take a bath (or give your kids one), do some gardening, listen to music, read a book, do the cooking – anything to allow your mind to switch off and your body to take a break. By the time the transition activity is over, you will be relaxed enough to begin looking forward to later love-making.

Keeping Moving

It's obvious that taking regular exercise will help you to stay energetic and enthusiastic during a lengthy session of love-making, and that it will tone you up and make you look good in bed. What may not be so obvious is that exercise keeps your body working to full potential. Exercise strengthens the heart for longer-lasting exertion, staves off heart attacks, hypertension and other sex-affecting illnesses. It makes nerve disorders less likely, and hormonal flow more effective.

The bottom line is that in order to keep healthy and sexually at your peak, you need to take the following exercise each week.

- **Exercise for suppleness.** Daily movement of your limbs and waist, joints and muscles: e.g., walking, Do It Yourself, housework, gardening, most sport, dancing.

- **Exercise for strength.** Lifting a heavy weight for at least five seconds daily: e.g., lifting furniture, shopping or children, heavy gardening, any work that involves manual labour.

- **Exercise for muscles and bones.** Being on your feet for at least two hours a day: e.g., walking, housework, any activity that involves standing.

- **Exercise for getting blood flow moving and heartbeat raised.** Twenty minutes vigorous activity for every second day: e.g., dancing, vigorous sport, brisk walking, playing with children.

- **Exercise for specifically sexual muscles.** Practising pelvic exercises daily so as to enable you to last longer and intensify your orgasm; these exercises are described below.

Be careful not to jump immediately into very strenuous exercise: use gentle stretching for a few minutes beforehand to warm up and afterwards to wind down. Sprained backs do not a good sex life make. In fact, if you are over forty, not in regular training or not in good health, we would advise you to cut out any energetic exercise you are already doing and work back up to a strenuous regime more slowly.

Pelvic Exercises

First developed by yoga masters thousands of years ago to improve sexual control and make orgasm even better, these exercises strengthen your pelvic muscles, increase the blood flow to your pelvic organs and help you focus your attention on genital sensation during sex.

Begin by practising when you are urinating, stopping the flow. When you are at ease with doing this, learn to stop the flow without using your stomach muscles – put your hand over your tummy to make sure you are not cheating.

Then, practise the same movement when not urinating, tightening and relaxing your pelvic muscles. Build up your strength so that you can hold the tightening movement for a few seconds.

Practise anywhere, at your desk, the bus stop, at home. Link it in to something you do regularly, such as eating or cleaning your teeth, so that you end up doing it several times a day

Action Plan

How can you change your lifestyle to one that will better support your sexuality? The key is not to go overboard, giving up everything except low-calorie coleslaw. Rather, look at what you already do, notice what you are already getting right, and slowly and gently shift to a better way of living.

Let us first summarize the total hit list:

- say yes to fresh, high-fibre, low-fat, low-sugar and low-salt foods;
- say no to processed, low-fibre, high-fat food, sugar, salt, and stimulants;
- discover and avoid any foods to which you might be sensitive;
- eat at the right time of day for you;
- eat only as much as you need to maintain weight and health;
- make sure your vitamin and mineral intake is adequate;
- make sure your alcohol consumption is within limits;
- give up smoking;
- regulate your use of drugs;
- get the right kind of sleep;
- relax regularly; and
- take the right kind of exercise.

Now the action plan.

1. For seven days, keep a diary, in a notebook you can take with you wherever you go. Write down everything you eat, drink or inhale, with the amount and the time. Don't just write 'potatoes...', write 'a large portion of chips, 2.30'; don't just write 'drinks...', write 'a double gin and tonic, 7.00'. If you notice yourself feeling odd after eating certain foods at certain times, note this down, too. Notice when you go to bed, how long you sleep, how you feel when you wake. Learn to notice when, during each day, you feel tense or relaxed. Work out just what you already do in the way of exercise.

2. After a week, look closely at what your patterns are and what changes you need to make in order to have a body that is fit for sex. You may want to:

- increase some things (unprocessed food, vitamin intake, length of sleep, relaxation time, amount of exercise);
- decrease some things (fatty foods, sugar, the total amount you eat, stimulants, alcohol, length of sleep, tension-creating occasions);
- cut out some things completely (food you may be allergic to, cigarettes); and
- change the nature of some things (eat at different times of day, go to bed earlier or later; alter your exercise schedule).

3. Choose one change (cutting down on your drinking, for example). Find the answers to all these questions, about that change, in order to motivate you.

- Why should I change? (Drinking is giving me brewer's droop.)
- What is blocking me from changing to my new lifestyle? (Friends might mock me.)
- How could I get round these blocks? (Order low-alcohol without them noticing.)
- What benefits do I get from sticking to my old lifestyle? (The social contact of drinking.)
- How could I replace these benefits in some way? (Find other social situations where drink isn't so important.)

4. Bearing in mind your answers to these questions, brainstorm a list of actions you could take to make your change. Sample ideas might be:

Food. *Omit.* If you always choose hamburger at lunchtime because there is nothing else available in the canteen, take a packed lunch instead.

Replace. Many foods have healthier alternatives: use oven chips in place of deep-fried, diet colas in place of high-sugar ones.

Prepare differently. Grill rather than fry; steam vegetables rather than boiling all the Vitamin C out of them.

Reduce your intake. Take half portions, eat more slowly; it takes twenty minutes for the signals of fullness to travel from stomach to brain.

Drink. *Replace.* Low- and non-alcoholic drinks are no longer seen as a coward's way out.

Delay. Stick to non-alcoholic drinks until half an hour before closing time and you will automatically drink less.

Extend the gaps. Alternate day on and day off, finding places other than the pub to go at lunchtime or in the evenings.

Smoking. Really, the only way is to *give up*. Don't do this at the same time as making any other changes to your diet or drinking regime – giving up smoking is enough to cope with on its own.

Drugs. As with smoking, any use of hard drugs has to *stop*. You may want to *control* your use of legal soft drugs as you would your drinking, by leaving long gaps between use.

Sleep. *Add inducements.* A good book to read before you drop off, a loving partner waiting for you in bed.

Take away temptation. Video tape good late-night films to prevent you staying up beyond your natural bedtime.

Add extra help. A herbal relaxant such as chamomile, a milky drink (but not stimulating cocoa or coffee) or a warm bath. Buy yourself a sleep tape which will talk you into slumber.

Relaxation. *Get a stress monitor.* Ask family or colleagues to spot and signal when body language shows you are tense.

Exercise. *Check your motivation factor.* Make sure you are taking exercise that is integrated with your life.

Work round the blocks. Use activities without equipment if you have none; exercise to the accompaniment of TV if you get bored.

5. Next, enrol help. Making even small changes will almost certainly mean your family will be involved. If it seems hard to do this, remember that your partner is likely to know already about the pros and cons of various foods and drinks, and will probably heave a sigh of relief if you ask her to join you in a healthier lifestyle.

6. Look at your list and choose just two small changes you can make over the next two weeks (order non-alcoholic drinks only; go bowling instead of to the pub on Tuesdays). After two weeks, make another two changes, and so on. Within just a few months you will have created a new lifestyle.

7. If you still find that changes you want to make have failed to stick, then think again. Particularly, if you are trying to crack the real biggies – giving up smoking, cutting down on alcohol, losing weight, starting to jog – then you may need extra help. Enrol colleagues, go to a support group, arrange to ring a friend if you start to renege. Remember that your whole sex life may be at stake.

8. If you are actually addicted – be that to drink, cigarettes or drugs – this is a big challenge, and not one this book can address. Appendix B lists many excellent organizations who know exactly what the challenges are and can help you meet them.

Addictions apart, however, the guidelines in this chapter will bring you to a level of physical health that will allow you to begin to contact your potential for Supervirility.

Looking Good and Getting Close

What your body looks like from the outside is just as important to Supervirility as how it functions on the inside. If you are in a long-term partnership, you probably won't be dressing to seduce – but you should still be thinking carefully about the way you use your body to attract. We are not trying to tell you how to dress, nor to persuade you to behave in a manner that isn't really you. What we are doing is offering some thoughts on how to use your physical presence to arouse. For nothing is more arousing, even for a partner who has known you for years, than looking good, smelling wonderful and moving well.

Looking Good

Given that you can't radically alter what Nature has given you, there is still a great deal you can do to present the basic package well. As mentioned in Chapter 2, keep slim, fit and well-toned. One of the two things that most turn a partner off over the years is a bulging tum landing on top of her in bed. (In case you're wondering, the other is bad breath.)

Men, as well as women, should keep their skin soft and supple. There is nothing unmasculine about using a barrier cream, all over if necessary, to ward off the effects of the weather or the central heating. Equally, use a good shampoo and conditioner on your hair. If you are balding, flaunt it; don't drape one piece over in a last-ditch stand!

Pay attention to detail. Keep your nails trimmed, as well as your beard and moustache. Get rid of nose or ear hair as soon as you spot it. Hairstyles do change, and so should yours. If you need an update, choose a local unisex hairdresser and insist on seeing one of the staff stylists, who won't be gone when you turn up for your next appointment in two months' time. Choose a hairdresser who looks neither too young and trendy, nor too old and staid. Talk through at length what you need and if, once it's done, you don't like it, ask for a recut in a few weeks' time. Keep going until you find a stylist who suits, then hang on to him or her like grim death for as long as you can!

Dressing up

If you want to be thought Supervirile, you should never dress to a macho image. Tight jeans and hairy chests are a man's idea of sexual prowess, but they are not most women's idea. Most women would rather have affection as a prelude to passion. Dress in soft, warm colours that suit you, in textures that invite hugs, and in styles that show your personality.

Colour co-ordination in clothes does make the most of what you wear. It means that everything you put on matches and looks planned; it will appeal to the majority of women who are very visually orientated, and who also work hard to co-ordinate their outfits. Colour assessment, when a consultant tests out which colours suit you and then prescribes a range from which you choose, may sound like a luxury, but can save you a fortune in wasted purchases that simply don't suit.

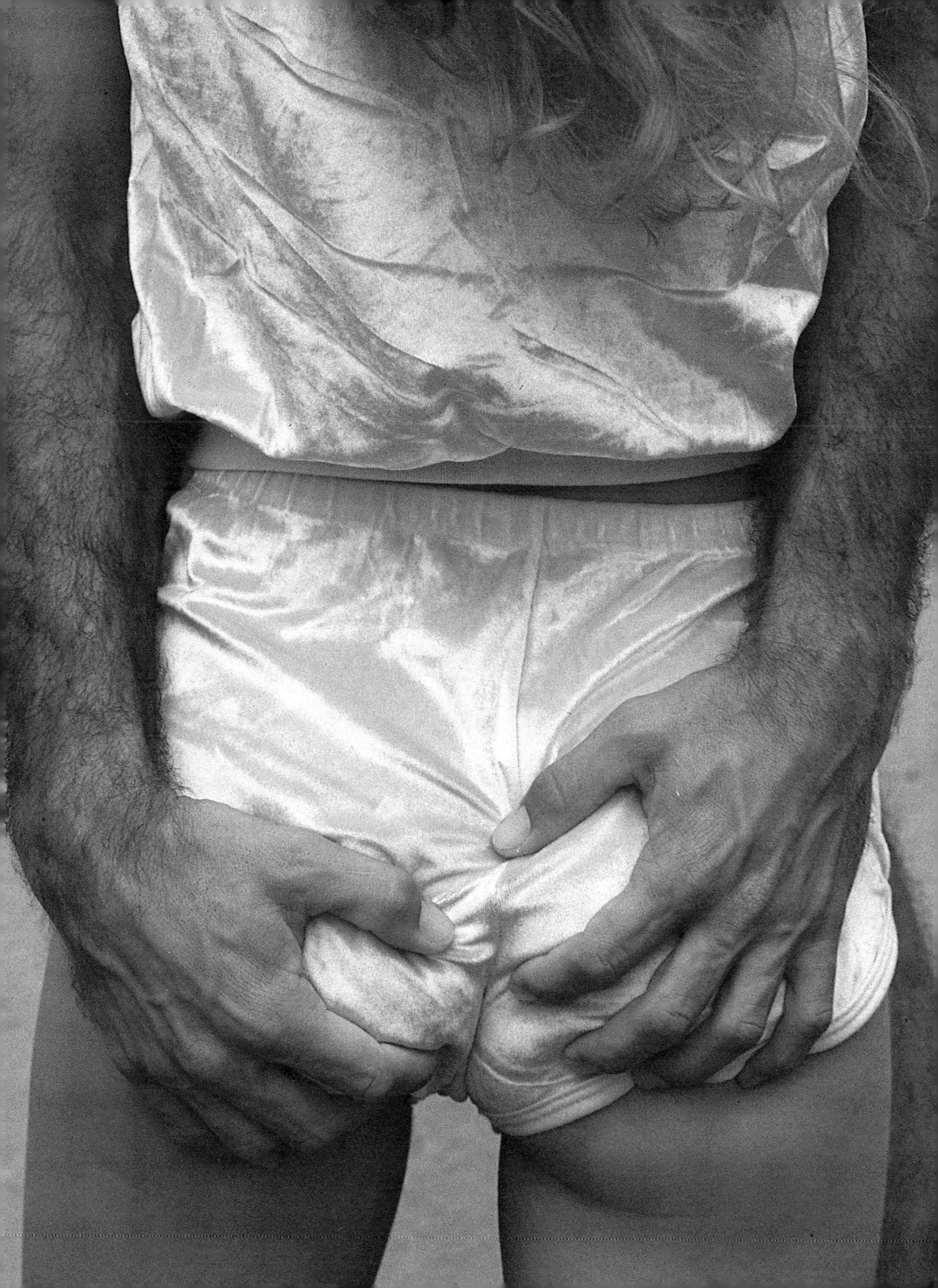

Dressing in high fashion only works if you have the money to keep rigorously abreast of trends. Conversely, don't let your image get out-of-date, wearing what you wore in 1973 because it makes you feel young. Dress from good, upmarket shops, buy fewer clothes than you think you should and pay more for them than you think you ought. Weed your wardrobe regularly, at least twice a year, and be ruthless.

To assess when you need an update, keep a weather eye on clothes magazines, even though you probably can't afford what they show. (It was estimated that readers of a leading men's magazine would have to be earning in excess of £70,000 per year to afford the outfits they were featuring!) If your partner has an eye for what suits you, take her with you on one or two shopping trips and watch how she chooses things; when you next shop alone, make the decisions you think she would make.

If you opt for a total change of image, go slowly. Make just one change at a time and give others and yourself time to adjust. If you do something dramatic as a result of reading this book, such as shaving off your beard or buying new underwear, reassure your partner that it isn't because you have just taken a lover!

SOUNDING GOOD

Don't fret if you don't like your voice; a noticeable accent or speech disorder may embarrass you, but to your partner it is part of the package. Your voice is a key ingredient of what she fell in love with, so don't be tempted to change it.

One way to continue to show your love and respect for a partner is to offer your partner equality in conversation. Men tend to think that, by talking a great deal, they are impressing their loved ones; this is a male myth. Women like to have their turn, to have their menfolk pause and allow them to speak, invite them into the conversation, ask questions and listen attentively.

There are ways to use your voice that will ease her into an affectionate mood. In general, seductive voices are ones that most reflect how we talk when we are feeling sexy; a low voice will invite your partner to come closer, a slow voice will invite relaxation, setting the mood for getting in touch with her feelings.

Also think of the emotion you can show in your voice. Don't try to pretend because it will seem false. But if you are feeling loving, let that show in your voice tone; and if you are feeling passionate, let that come through as you speak.

GETTING CLOSE

As you move closer to your partner, other senses than sight and sound come into play. Our bodies secrete chemicals that in animals are known to trigger sexual arousal. These communicate our sexual excitement, while turning our partner on. So don't bother with artificial smells such as aftershave. The best aphrodisiac you have at your disposal is your own natural smell.

Washing daily is therefore an essential part of allowing sexual links to grow between you. Allowing your natural smell to get masked by daily dirt means that she will be unable to receive the sexual messages you are sending. Wash with a mild or unscented soap all over, particularly your underarms, genitals (including under your foreskin if not circumcised) and feet.

As mentioned before, bad breath is a total anathema to sexual attractiveness, so make sure your dentist gets to see you regularly and that you do what is necessary with the toothbrush after each meal! If you find suddenly that your smell is not inviting to your partner, nor hers to you, ask yourself why. Eating unusual food, drinking heavily, ill health – or bad feeling in the relationship – can all influence how you communicate on this essential and often unconscious level. As semi-vegetarians, we personally find that a single meat meal can make us smell totally different to one another in bed!

Looking Good and Getting Close

Moving Together

The non-verbal communication of movement and touch that you have with your partner is the final piece in the jigsaw of how you express your sexuality to each other. The way you interact in terms of body language not only encourages or discourages your partner to have sex with you on any particular occasion. It also makes statements about your relationship that make it more, or less, likely that sex between you will blossom.

Be aware of the distance you and your partner like to be from each other at any particular time. Bridging the gap before she is ready – perhaps while she is winding down from work and settling into being at home in the evening – may feel invasive to her. Steering clear of her when she wants to touch may feel like rejection.

Equally, let your gestures to your partner, whether in public or private, be welcoming rather than excluding. Open gestures that leave your body unprotected are a sign of trust and wanting to enfold her; closed gestures across your body shut her out. When you both use the same kind of movements, with the same speed, rhythm and gesture, then you are feeling close to one another; read this as a signal that you can take the next step towards contact. Which is, perhaps, to let your eyes meet.

Long-time partners often avoid eye contact because they are with each other so much of the time they feel they don't need it. To reinstate the romance of your early years, try affectionate glances across the room when in public, and take the opportunity to have long, direct, intimate eye contact at home or in the semi-privacy of a dimly lit restaurant.

Between you, over the years or months, you will have built up a series of intimate codes which are special to you. Perhaps they involve brief glances, perhaps passing smiles. A tone of voice, a code word or a particular touch as you pass – all of these are the ways that you have developed between you of showing you care.

To fully meet what your partner wants of you, to create the right setting for true Super-virility, be aware of these codes and use them. Remember that a key aphrodisiac, even in a long-term relationship, is the knowledge that you are communicating in your own private language, and that what you are saying is 'I love you'.

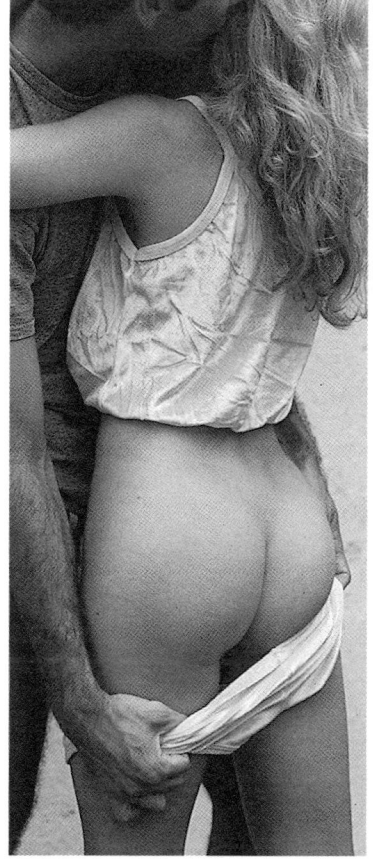

WHEN ILLNESS STRIKES

4

However much you work on your health and fitness, you are sometimes going to fall ill – and that can dramatically affect your sexuality. We personally have heard at least one horror story of a whole relationship breaking down because of illness-based problems – a fact that was only discovered *after* the divorce!

This chapter is one to skim. It is a reference source to use during illness, to track down any possible effects on your sexuality; also, if your sexuality is currently not what you want, use this chapter to check whether your health could be at fault. Incidentally, if you have a medical condition that has been known to lead to a sexual disorder, then don't assume you will be affected; the illnesses we mention often create problems for only a few sufferers. Desire is a vulnerable thing; if you believe that your illness will make you less than virile, then it will.

If you are one of the minority of men who have never been able to have an erection, or ejaculate, then this chapter will be especially relevant to you, as your condition is likely to be physical. However, as we mentioned in the Introduction, this book cannot deal with these issues in detail; see your doctor immediately.

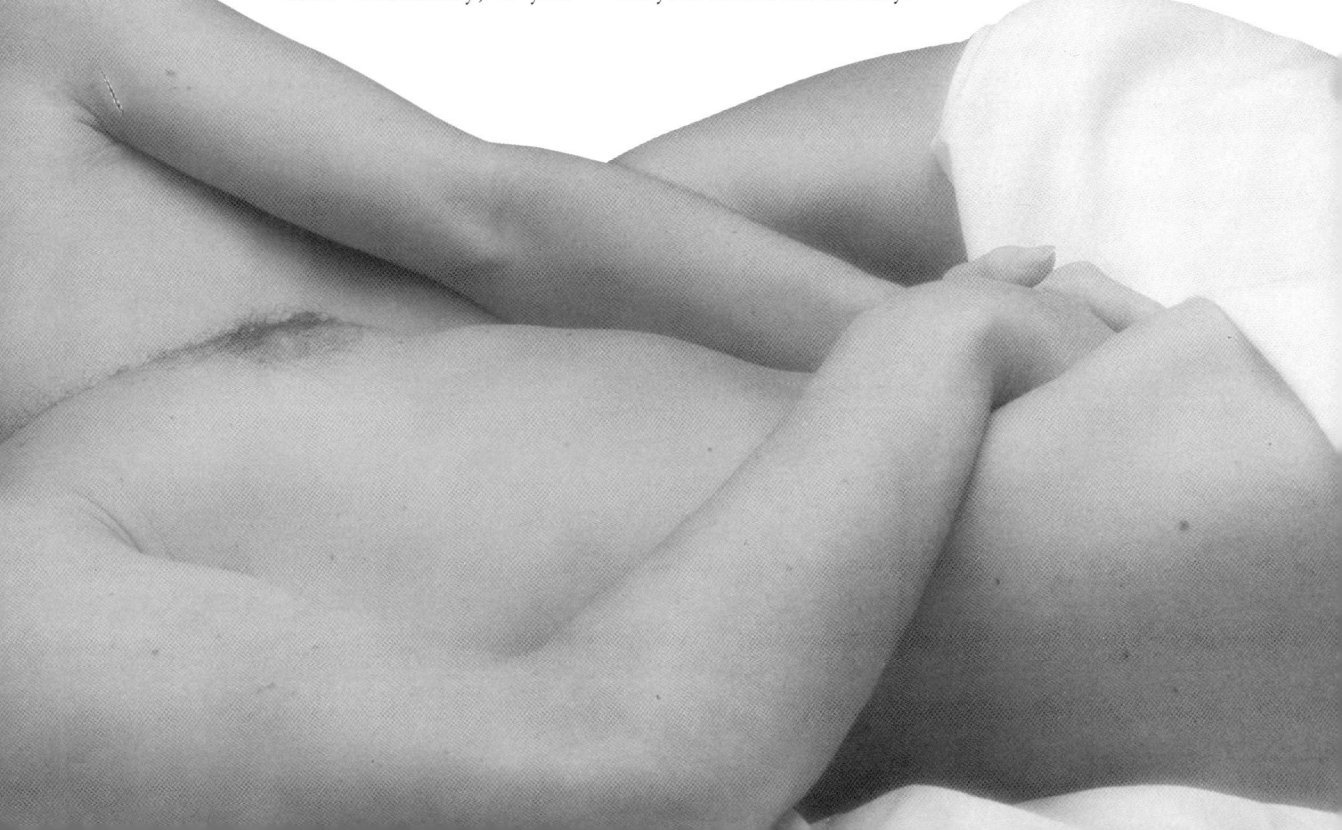

BODYWORKS – NOT WORKING

Any condition where you have difficulty in sexual movement, or feel anxious about exerting yourself will make you unenthusiastic about sex. One of the commonest is **Peyrnonies disease**, where hard patches of tissue on the penis make it seem curved when erect. Equally, your **foreskin** may be causing discomfort by being too tight, getting torn or developing an infection. Ask your doctor for minor surgery or stitching, and for antibiotics to cure infection.

Arthritis, which is not just a old man's disease, but strikes three year olds, causes stiff or painful joints, hardly conducive to swinging from the chandeliers. Choose a time of day for love-making when you feel least pain, take a hot bath beforehand, and experiment with positions until you find one that suits you best. A **heart attack** can leave you convinced that you may never dare make love again. But if you take things carefully, and check out with your doctor first, there is no reason for you not to resume sex quite soon: masturbate first to get your confidence up, and choose easy positions and a slow pace. If you are **disabled**, seek practical advice on how best to make love given the physical challenges you have. And seek emotional help on how to overcome any hesitation you may have about developing your sexuality. Make contact with a support group such as SPOD (Appendix B).

Some illnesses also make sex less attractive because they cause pain, discomfort and embarrassment in sexual parts of the body. They don't undermine your sexuality directly, but do interfere with it indirectly and psychologically. **Bladder problems** can be controlled by cutting down late-night drinks and irritant foods; **piles and haemmorhoids** can be treated with ointments. The **ostomies**, operations that mean you need to use a bag for holding urine or faeces, may create embarrassing difficulties. The sexual act itself is physically possible, but you need to time love-making for when your bag is empty and likely to remain so for some time; to make sure the bag fits well and doesn't leak; to choose a sexual position that takes the bag into account. A sympathetic partner is worth her weight in gold here!

A final 'bodyworks' problem is when the **prostate gland** may over time enlarge and block the passing of urine. This in itself is no problem. But, if you need surgery, this sometimes makes you unable to ejaculate; there are usually no side-effects applying specifically to erection or orgasm, so you end up with the sensation but not the fluid. It's a worry, but not a problem, unless of course you want to start a family. Luckily this condition usually only strikes older men for whom this is less likely to be an issue.

WHEN BLOOD FLOW DROPS

Good sexuality needs good blood flow, particularly into the penis. Difficulty with erection may alert you to **hardening of the arteries** or to **high blood pressure**, both of which affect penile blood flow. All the food and exercise hints we gave in Chapter 3 will help prevention and, if you do develop either condition, your doctor will help with medication – though check that this medication itself is not affecting your desire levels.

One particular blood-flow disorder is the **venous leak**. When arousal begins, blood flows into the penis through arteries, and then veins dilate to prevent blood from flowing out. When the blood does not go into the erectile tissue, but flows straight out again, then erection simply doesn't happen. This condition can sometimes be corrected with surgery.

Kidney disease, with its impact on the effectiveness of the blood, often causes loss of interest and erectile difficulties. If you do have kidney problems, your doctor will be

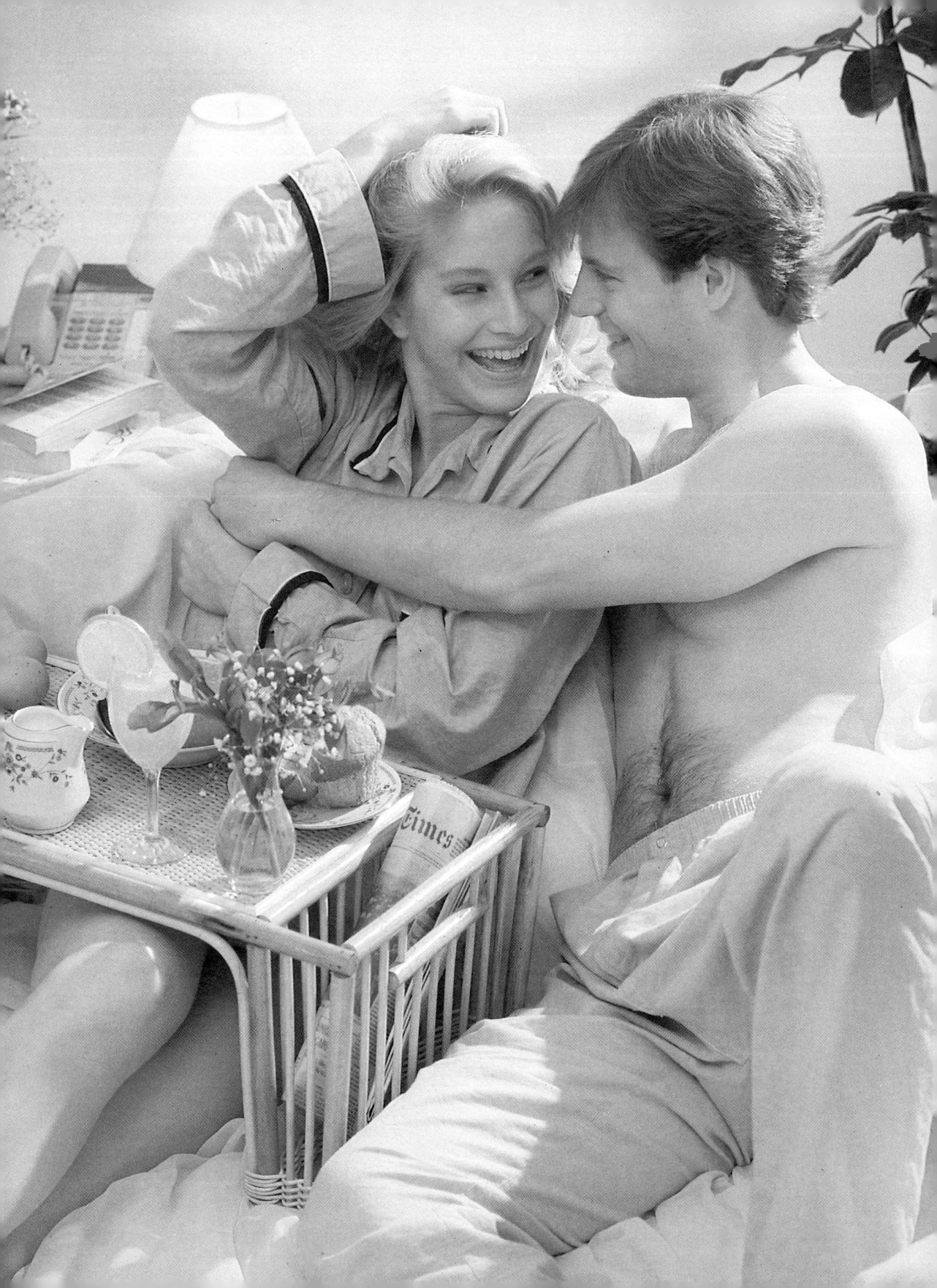

able to advise the best approach for you to take; it may also be useful to make sure you are getting enough zinc in your diet, as the blood 'cleaning' necessary in kidney dialysis may deplete zinc stores vital to sexual functioning. A kidney transplant may help by giving you back normal blood function.

BRAIN POWER AND NERVE NUISANCES

As the brain is the control centre of our desire, any condition which disturbs the brain will also disturb your sexuality. **Brain tumours, stress, depression, drugs** and **alcohol** all affect your brain and hence your love-making. Follow your doctor's direction as to treatment and, if relevant, check that your medication isn't making the situation worse (see page 44).

Diabetes, from an imbalance of insulin in the body, is particularly likely to cause erectile difficulties through nerve damage; in fact, sudden impotence can be the first warning sign of diabetes. If you find yourself losing weight, drinking vast amounts of liquid and urinating frequently, then get your blood sugar level checked by your doctor. If caught early, and the insulin imbalance restored by correct diet and injection, diabetes need not have long-term effects.

Multiple sclerosis attacks the nerve fibres all over the body. In the early stages you may get diminished sensation in your penis and pelvic area, or not be able to get aroused by thinking alone; use direct stimulation by yourself or your partner for the desired effect. In the long term, serious deterioration of the nerves through MS may mean serious effects on your sexuality.

Spinal or pelvic injuries or operations can spoil both erection and ejaculation by damaging the nervous system. You may need to be creative in how you get and maintain an erection, using hands, mouth and sex toys. The good news is that there have been reports of other parts of the body increasing in sensitivity to compensate for nerve loss.

WHEN HORMONES FADE

One particular and currently controversial physical problem has particular relevance to Supervirility – hormone imbalance. Problems with these chemical messengers that stimulate sexual behaviour will obviously create difficulties. Unfortunately, our knowledge of hormones is still so primitive that scientists are not quite sure how they work. There certainly has to be enough testosterone for erection to take place normally, and it is probably safe to say that low testosterone affects sex drive, too. Castrated men do suffer loss of desire, as may men whose testosterone-producing glands have become infected or are unusually small. High stress and steady drinking create a drop in hormone levels, although these levels may return to normal once the pressure is off.

So far, no argument. Where the medical profession does disagree is whether there is a natural drop in testosterone as men get older. Women have a midlife drop in hormone levels – but do men? Some experts argue that, as most men, unlike women, continue to produce testosterone throughout their lives, there is no comparison; that men with erectile difficulties often seem to have perfectly normal hormone levels when tested; that true hormone deficiency is not all that common. These experts offer replacement therapy to patients only in situations where low hormone levels are truly measurable.

Other experts believe that it is worthwhile looking at a body's ability to use what testosterone it has, rather than simply at measurable levels. Dr Malcolm Carruthers, the current champion of hormone treatment in Britain, points out that men may have different thresholds of testosterone needed for sexual desire, so perhaps even a slight drop may be taking you just below the level you require for sex drive and erection. He believes in what he calls the male viropause (like the female menopause), particularly following vasectomy, and suggests 'giving Nature a helping hand' by supplementing with natural testosterone.

If you suspect you have a hormone imbalance then check with your doctor. On page 51 we look in more detail at how hormone therapy might help.

TAKING THE TABLETS

No medical drug always has sexual side-effects, but some have been known to cause difficulties for up to twenty-five per cent of men taking them. If you are suffering from any of the following diseases, it is worthwhile getting your doctor to check whether the medication he is prescribing has any published side-effects. If so, ask whether you can have alternative medication, stop medication or take any of the treatments we suggest in brackets.

- **Cancer.** Some hormone-based medication affects sexuality.

- **Cardiac failure.** Digoxin can cause loss of desire.

- **Depression.** A range of drugs can cause erection difficulties or delayed ejaculation (try psychotherapy, or complementary medicine such as acupuncture or homoeopathy).

- **Epilepsy.** Some anti-convulsants cause loss of desire.

- **Glaucoma.** Some drugs cause delayed ejaculation.

- **Hardening of the arteries** and **high blood pressure.** Many patients have in the past had delayed ejaculation; new drugs are less problematic (try relaxation techniques, diet, acupuncture, homoeopathy).

- **Muscle development.** Steroids used for weight gain in sports can alter your hormone balance.

- **Pain.** Morphine-based painkillers sometimes disrupt erection (try acupuncture).

- **Sleep problems.** Some sleeping tablets affect libido and erection (try relaxation techniques and meditation).

- **Spastic colon.** Some drugs can cause delayed ejaculation.

- **Tension.** Sedatives dull the senses (try relaxation techniques or meditation).

- **Ulcers.** Medication can cause poor erections and delayed ejaculation.

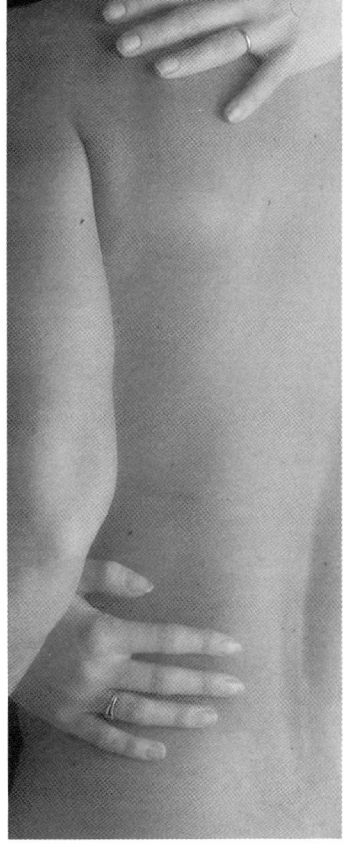

Sexual Nasties

If you or your partner develop a sexually transmitted disease (STD), then you have opened a Pandora's box of both practical and emotional blocks to sexual fulfilment. Here is a brief guide to symptoms, causes and treatment.

- **Non-specific urethritis.** Warning signs include discharge and burning on passing urine. Not necessarily sexually transmitted. Drink lots of water, take rest, see doctor for medication.

- **Trichomoniasis.** Few warning signs; possibly a thin, yellow-green discharge. Not necessarily sexually transmitted. Drink lots of water, see a doctor for medication.

- **Crabs.** Nits or eggs appearing on hair or clothes. Transmitted by any close contact. Use an over-the-counter lotion or shampoo.

- **Warts.** Small bumps on penis and genitals. Probably passed sexually, but can develop years after initial contact. See doctor for ointment, or burning under local anaesthetic.

- **Chlamydia.** Burning on urination and creamy discharge. Transmitted by sexual contact. See doctor for antibiotics.

- **Herpes.** Painful open sores. Not necessarily sexually transmitted. No known treatment; self-help includes pain-killers, ice packs and wearing loose trousers. You are infectious well before the symptoms show.

- **Gonorrhoea** ('the clap'). Burning pain on urination, pus-like discharge. Passed sexually, and can rear its head in oral and anal versions. Treatment is usually a single dose of penicillin, but a follow-up test is vital.

- **Syphilis.** A painless open sore followed by a non-itchy rash. Once spotted, treatable with antibiotics. If not spotted, can be fatal in the end. It is rare.

- **HIV (human immunodeficiency virus).** Passed through exchange of the body fluids: blood, semen, vaginal and cervical secretions and probably breast milk (not saliva, sweat, urine or tears). It can't be passed through whole, scabbed or covered skin – but unscabbed cuts will make you vulnerable. **HIV** destroys important cells within the immune system, leaving people with reduced immunity to a range of infections and diseases, some of which may prove fatal. Many people with **HIV** infection who have become seriously ill are said to have AIDS (acquired immune deficiency syndrome).

Some experts now advise the use of condoms even if you are in a long-term relationship where other contraception is being used, because, properly used, the condom is a largely effective barrier against **HIV** and a range of other more common **STDs**.

If you think you have any form of STD, go to your doctor or clinic immediately; consultation and treatment are free and usually extremely sympathetic. Use condoms right away to protect your partner from infection, and you from re-infection. She should get a check-up, too; many infections have more serious consequences for women than for men.

You must talk things through with your partner. Often, the causes of infection are non-sexual, or stem from relationships well before you met – but the implications for your partnership, and therefore for your sexuality, need to be faced. All the skills we suggest you need in a sexually fulfilling relationship (see Part III) are even more vital here if you are to turn what seems like a problem into an opportunity.

5 Body Help

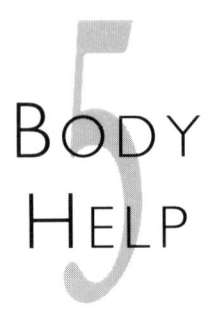

What now? Perhaps as a by-product of illness, you have a sexual block which can only be solved with medical help. Or perhaps, though you are not ill, you feel that only outside intervention can give you the sexuality you deserve. This chapter outlines some routes that you might choose to take.

First Checks

The first step in beginning to get extra support for your body is to do three simple checks.

**Check one –
is it your body that needs extra help?**

Many blocks to sexuality are nothing to do with your body functioning. If you wonder whether your attitudes to sex or to your partner are really at issue, then check whether the sections on mind, relationship and sexual skill ring bells for you. In particular, if you can get hard, regular erections spontaneously or when you are masturbating, but the erection fails when with your partner, you should think again about whether your sexual blocks are really physical ones

**Check two –
are you suffering from a minor illness?**

Do you feel fine? Are you tired, irritable, have no energy, keep going down with minor colds or stomach upsets? If so, you are probably run down and it is not surprising that your body is not responding. You don't need specialist help. Go to the doctor if you need medication and, alongside this, eat well, get more vitamins, stop drinking alcohol or taking soft drugs for at least a week; sleep round the clock if you need to. Take time off and give your body a total break.

**Check three –
is your body sending you danger signals?**

These would include pain in the genitals; discharge of any kind; swellings in penis or testicles; obvious changes in your waterworks including blood; changes in semen including blood; change in your vision, smell or hearing; any small, hard, painless lumps on any part of your body. If you have any of these symptoms, if you cannot get an erection under any circumstances, or if you suddenly find yourself unable to ejaculate, go to your doctor right away rather than trying any of the self-help methods we suggest.

Getting Support

We look first at the range of possibilities you can buy to enhance or support your erection. These have a long pedigree, though we are wary, feeling they add to the myth that all love-making depends on erection, as well as potentially masking a deeper, underlying physical disorder that needs exploring. That said, these methods can be fun to use and are meant to allow you to carry on longer than you normally could – or to raise the dead when it is unwilling to raise itself. Also, if your penis has had an off-day in the past, these methods can give you the reassurance to try love-making again, getting back enough confidence not to sink into a failure spiral.

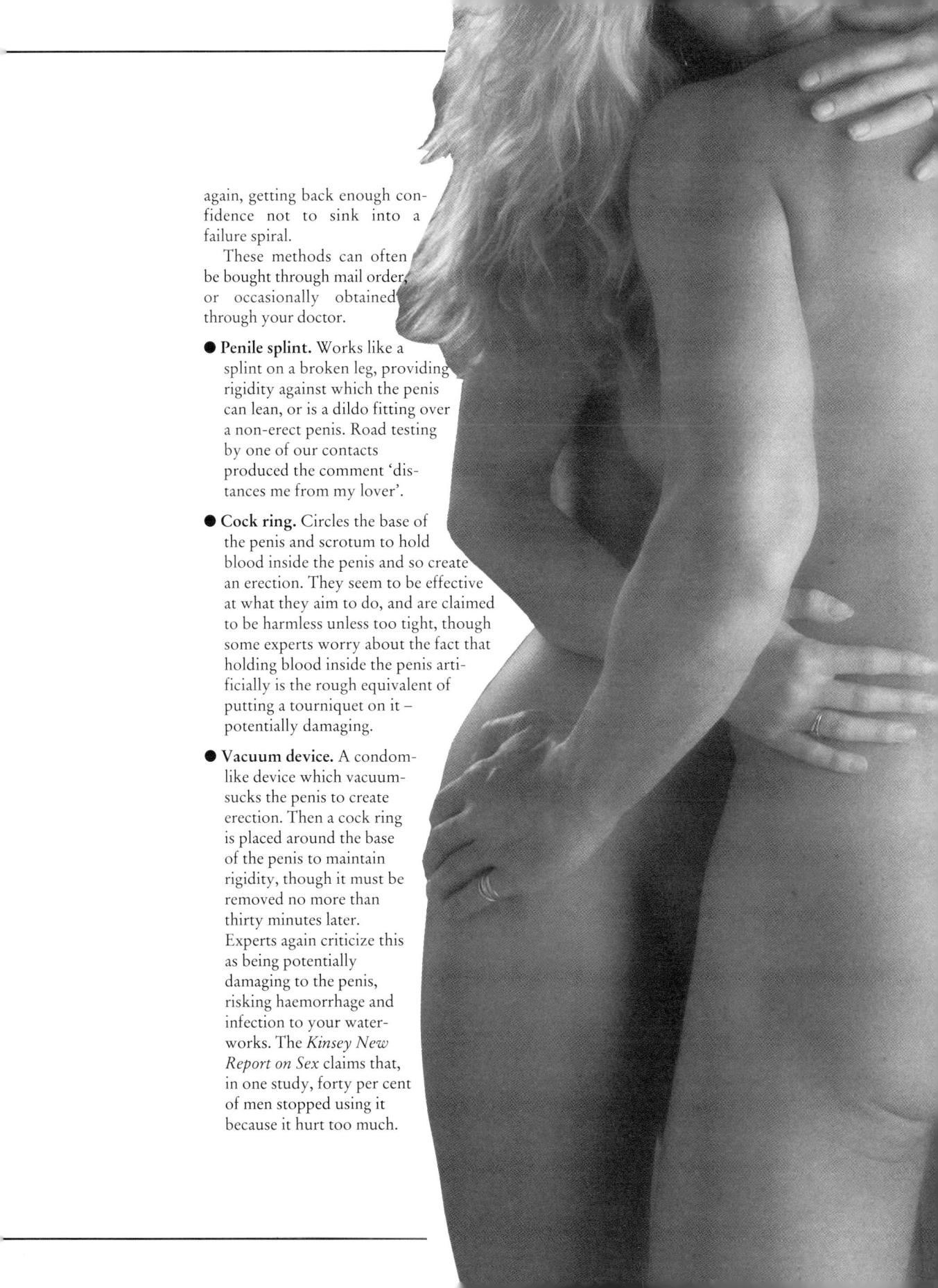

These methods can often be bought through mail order, or occasionally obtained through your doctor.

- **Penile splint.** Works like a splint on a broken leg, providing rigidity against which the penis can lean, or is a dildo fitting over a non-erect penis. Road testing by one of our contacts produced the comment 'distances me from my lover'.

- **Cock ring.** Circles the base of the penis and scrotum to hold blood inside the penis and so create an erection. They seem to be effective at what they aim to do, and are claimed to be harmless unless too tight, though some experts worry about the fact that holding blood inside the penis artificially is the rough equivalent of putting a tourniquet on it – potentially damaging.

- **Vacuum device.** A condom-like device which vacuum-sucks the penis to create erection. Then a cock ring is placed around the base of the penis to maintain rigidity, though it must be removed no more than thirty minutes later. Experts again criticize this as being potentially damaging to the penis, risking haemorrhage and infection to your waterworks. The *Kinsey New Report on Sex* claims that, in one study, forty per cent of men stopped using it because it hurt too much.

Classes and Courses

The next step in getting outside help may be to join some kind of course. Many of these are near to home; they provide a supportive environment which will encourage you to keep going – and any difficulties you have can be solved by your tutor or group leader.

- **Exercise classes.** These offer a way to get together with others if your motivation is low. Your local evening institute will have classes, as will your local health club – some clubs also run schemes whereby you train with an individual trainer.
- **Relaxation classes.** Often run at evening institutes or local health centres, these classes are also done by some large companies in-house. They are usually spread over two or three sessions, in which you learn mental and physical relaxation.
- **Massage.** Various forms can be learned alone or with your partner through classes at evening institutes, or through personal growth centres. Such classes increase sensual awareness and have a supportive environment in which to improve your body image. Back home, you can use your skills for sensual massage (see Chapter 16).
- **Biofeedback machines.** These machines tell you when you are tense – a key block to sensuality. Measuring devices on the palm of your hand or the tips of your fingers monitor tension through your skin response or temperature – and your body gradually learns what you need to do to relax. We have also heard (but have no first-hand reports) of penile biofeedback devices being used to help you gain control of your erection. Run by private organizations which charge fees, biofeedback courses may take several sessions.
- **Yoga.** An Eastern system of philosophy which in the West often concentrates on physical skills. Yoga is based around body movements, which are designed to exercise, increase flexibility and relax you. Although some Eastern sexuality manuals mention yoga exercises for enhancing love-making, we have yet to find a Western method that teaches these.

Complementary Help

The next step may be to try complementary medicine. Despite its name, complementary medicine is not only about curing symptoms, but also about raising health levels so that you can enjoy sex more.

Complementary practitioners usually practise outside the orthodox health systems. Find them by tracking down your local alternative health centre, looking in the phone book, or contacting a centralized organization which will then give you a list of practitioners in your area. Appendix B lists central organizations for the therapies we describe.

Of course, if you have a particular medical symptom, then check with your doctor that he or she is happy for you to have complementary treatment; most traditional practitioners recognize that complementary medicine does help, and most complementary practitioners are happy to do their bit alongside whatever standard medical treatment you're getting.

- **Acupuncture.** This therapy sees the body as having certain energy paths or meridians which can get blocked and need unblocking. Two main kinds of acupuncture are used in Britain and most of the Western World: both methods use needles and burning herbs to unblock the meridians, and both claim they can help with sexual blocks. Acupuncture treatments last up to an hour.

- **Alexander Technique.** This technique gained its current reputation as a way of solving back problems, but aims to re-align and maximize body use in all kinds of ways. It claims to resolve all sorts of sexual blocks such as premature ejaculation, as well as enhancing sex by making you more responsive.

- **Aromatherapy.** This therapy is based on the principle that essential plant oils affect your mood, your psyche and your physical state. Some oils, like ylang ylang and rose, are thought to increase your virility. Massage with essential oils can also be very sensuous. Or try lavender on the radiator or light bulb by your bed to experience complete relaxation. An aromatherapist will blend oils to suit your particular needs.

- **Homoeopathy.** Homoeopathy works on the principle that some substances which actually cause symptoms can, in small doses, push your body into building up its defences and curing itself. A homoeopath may prescribe liquids, pills or powders, probably only in single doses. All prescriptions take into consideration your character, state of mind, weaknesses and strengths. The prescribed substances will urge your body to do what is necessary to resolve sexual blocks.

TRADITIONAL HELP

You may still feel you need further help, and another alternative is to turn to traditional medical practitioners. However, first, a word of warning. Don't rush for the medical solution thinking that it will automatically solve your problem. It may not have the answer; there are no quick fixes, no magic wands. Firstly, for example, most traditional medical solutions are aimed at curing erectile difficulty, and have little to offer with other sexual vulnerabilities. Secondly, be aware that entirely physical solutions only work if it is entirely physical causes that are holding you back. If there are any mental or emotional causes, then they won't work – and, in fact, there are very few practitioners who will offer you only a physical solution. Whether you attend for surgery, drug treatment or hormone replacement therapy, you will almost certainly be asked to look at your current life as a whole.

The first thing to do if you suspect that only medical intervention will help is to go to your doctor; be prepared for him to ask you about these points:

- what you are worried about or what you want to change, when you became aware that you were worried or wanted things to change;

- what your physical patterns of sexuality are: how often you have a spontaneous erection, how often you masturbate, how often you have intercourse, how long intercourse lasts, how easy it is for you to come, how long it takes for you to feel sexual again; and

- your general health, particularly your patterns of smoking, alcohol, sleep, relaxation, exercise, medication, plus any tendency towards heart disease, hypertension, waterworks problems and nervous illness.

Your doctor will almost certainly give you a physical examination and some basic tests such as blood pressure and urine checks. He will wonder whether any physical cause for your sexual block falls into one of the following categories – and so he may have you checked by experts who will carry out tests.

- **Your nervous system.** A neurologist may check your brain, spinal cord, nerves and muscle responses; he may test your reflexes and ask you to monitor your night-time erection.

- **Your heart and blood flow.** A vascular consultant may check the workings of arteries and veins, which can be done by an ultrasound scan or by injecting drugs to assess blood flow round the body and particularly into your penis.

- **Your waterworks.** A urologist may examine your genitals, urinary system, kidneys and bladder.

- **Your hormone system.** An endocrinologist may do a series of blood tests to reveal your hormone level.

- **An insulin test.** May be done additionally as sudden loss of erectile function can be an early warning sign of diabetes.

Needless to say, these tests take time. While you are waiting for the results, you help yourself by working on nutrition, and relaxation. In particular, take regular exercise designed to strengthen your heart and lungs – swimming is ideal. That way, if an operation or medical procedure is necessary, your body will be ready for it.

When the results come through, it could be that your doctor will pronounce you medically fit, or indicate that he doesn't consider medical intervention appropriate. If you really believe he is wrong, ask for a second opinion; but don't just keep switching until you find someone who will treat you. There are charlatans around who, realizing that sex is one area where people will move heaven, earth and bank balances to get a result, offer treatment where none is actually necessary.

If treatment is the next stop, what kinds are on offer? We outline here, in some detail, the possibilities and how they can help.

SURGICAL OPTIONS

Where for one reason or another blood flow just simply doesn't create an erection, it is possible to have a penile implant to stiffen the penis, and this has no effect – bad or good – on ejaculation or orgasm.

The first kind of implant is an inflatable device, a pump-up cylinder which is surgically implanted in your penis, with tubing linking it to a fluid reservoir in your abdomen wall and a pump in your scrotum. When you need an erection, you pump fluid into your penis until it is erect enough; when the erection is no longer needed, you deflate it. This kind works well, though it is expensive. The second kind of implant consists of two inert rods which fill your penis, so that it is always erect. Though cheaper, it lacks the flexibility of the other kind of implant.

We tend to be wary of implant surgery because of the risk involved in any operation, and also because it permanently destroys any ability to get a natural erection. Equally, putting the emphasis on erection being the key element in lovemaking does worry us. And, it is certainly true that reports show the partners of men with implants being not quite as impressed with the solution as their husbands were. So check out fully with your partner before taking such a major step. But where erection does seem to be physically impossible, and where having an erection is really important to you and your partner, then an implant may be the answer.

DRUG OPTIONS

At the moment there are a very few prescribed drugs that affect sexual functioning with any reliability. If lack of blood flow into your penis is causing difficulty, then you may discuss with your doctor using blood-vessel-dilating drugs. If coming too soon is a problem, there are one or two anti-depressants that may help, but they have side-effects.

There is one exception to this, however – papaverine. We talked to Dr John Moran, who uses the drug as part of his sexual therapy practice. While the thought of injecting a drug directly into your penis may cause you to shiver, Dr Moran told us that papaverine has been proved to cause erections in most men – so that if you are suffering from erectile dysfunction, you can learn to dose yourself when needed. For many, this is a simple solution. There have been criticisms: some people are wary that papaverine treats only the symptoms, and point out that scientists have no idea of the long-term consequences of induced erections. But there are also many satisfied customers – and, as Dr Moran points out, 'The sheer fact that you know you can have an erection when you want one may take away any anxiety and so you may find that your natural erection comes back of its own accord.' The one exception to easy use of papaverine are those men who have blood-flow disorders – with them, it simply doesn't work.

HORMONE OPTIONS

If you are suffering from hormone deficiency, then there are two easy ways to top up your hormone levels: tablets and implants. Most doctors offer tablets for the first three to six months, and then check both whether your hormone levels have risen, and whether you are feeling more desire and are having more successful sex. If hormone therapy suits you, you can then go on to have pellets of fused testosterone crystals implanted in a small cut made in your buttocks.

It sounds painful, but when we 'observed' a cheerful client having it done, the local anaesthetic seemed to take all discomfort away, allowing him to lie happily on his tummy and chat to us while his doctor piled pellets into the not inconsiderable scalpel hole. This client reported a rise in virility, energy, vigour and general well-being. He had his implant renewed every six months, at which time a careful check was made to make sure he suffered no ill-effects.

Hormone treatment is currently very controversial. Doctors who test your hormone levels will offer to give you replacement therapy if they find your levels are below the optimal amount. If they don't find that, though, they may argue that you don't need extra hormones and that extra hormones may create medical problems.

On the other hand, Dr Malcolm Carruthers, in whose surgery the above-mentioned implant took place, claims that this is simply the medical establishment suffering from a severe case of sour grapes – such as it suffered when female hormone replacement therapy was first mooted. He champions the use of hormone therapy for lowered stress, raised energy and general Supervirility rather than just to create erection, and cites research showing many satisfied customers and minimal side-effects.

If you feel that your blocks may be due to hormone imbalance, then there are certainly things you can do if you are refused hormone therapy. First, make sure that you are keeping fit, keeping stress levels low and, in particular, cutting down on alcohol which drops your testosterone level. Secondly, remember that there is some evidence that sex keeps hormone levels high – so turn your attention to doing it more, and more pleasurably, and as often as you and your partner want to. After that, it is up to you whether you trust the current state of research sufficiently to be prepared to fight for, and often pay for, extra help.

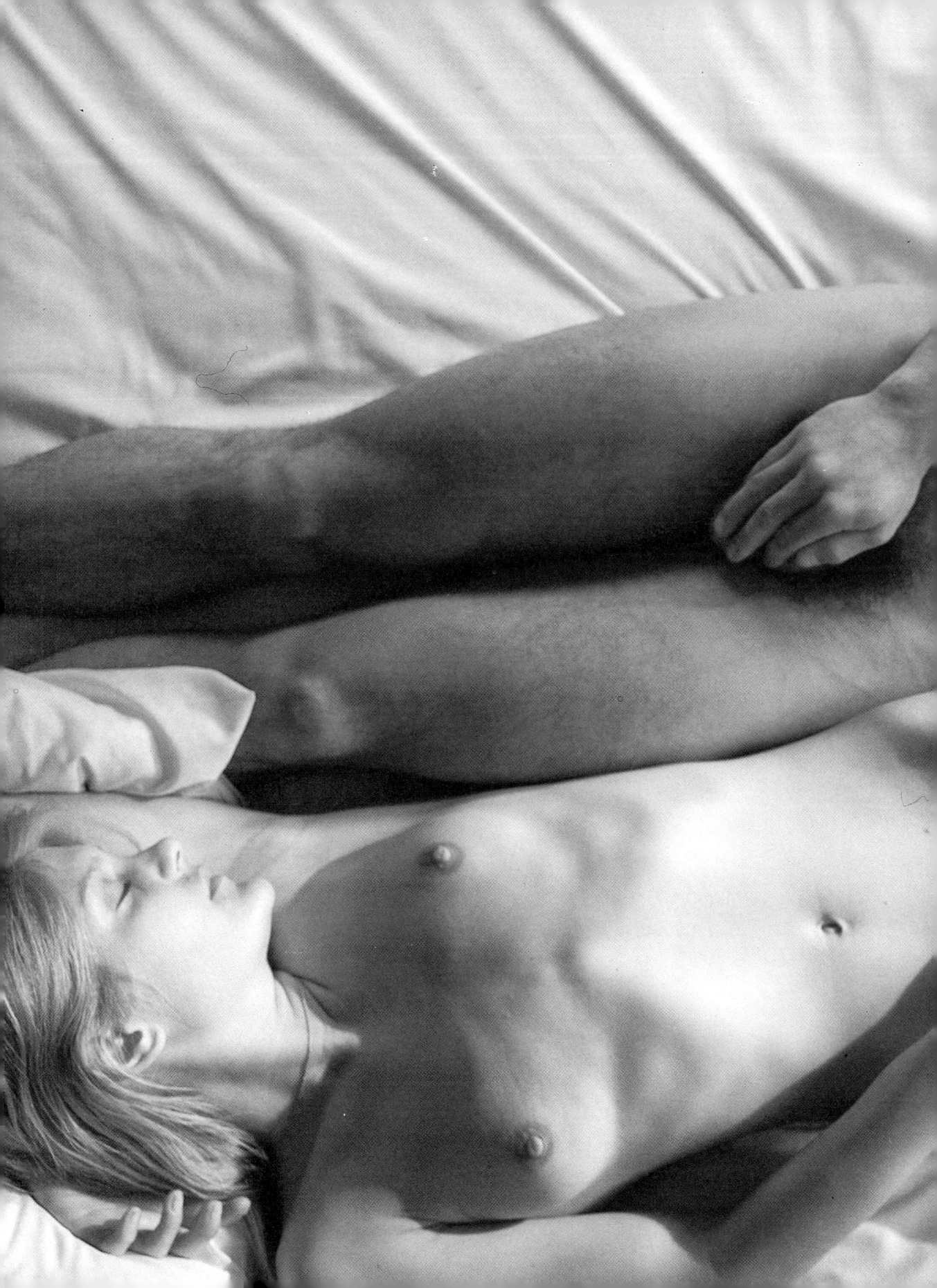

Part II
Mind Supervirility

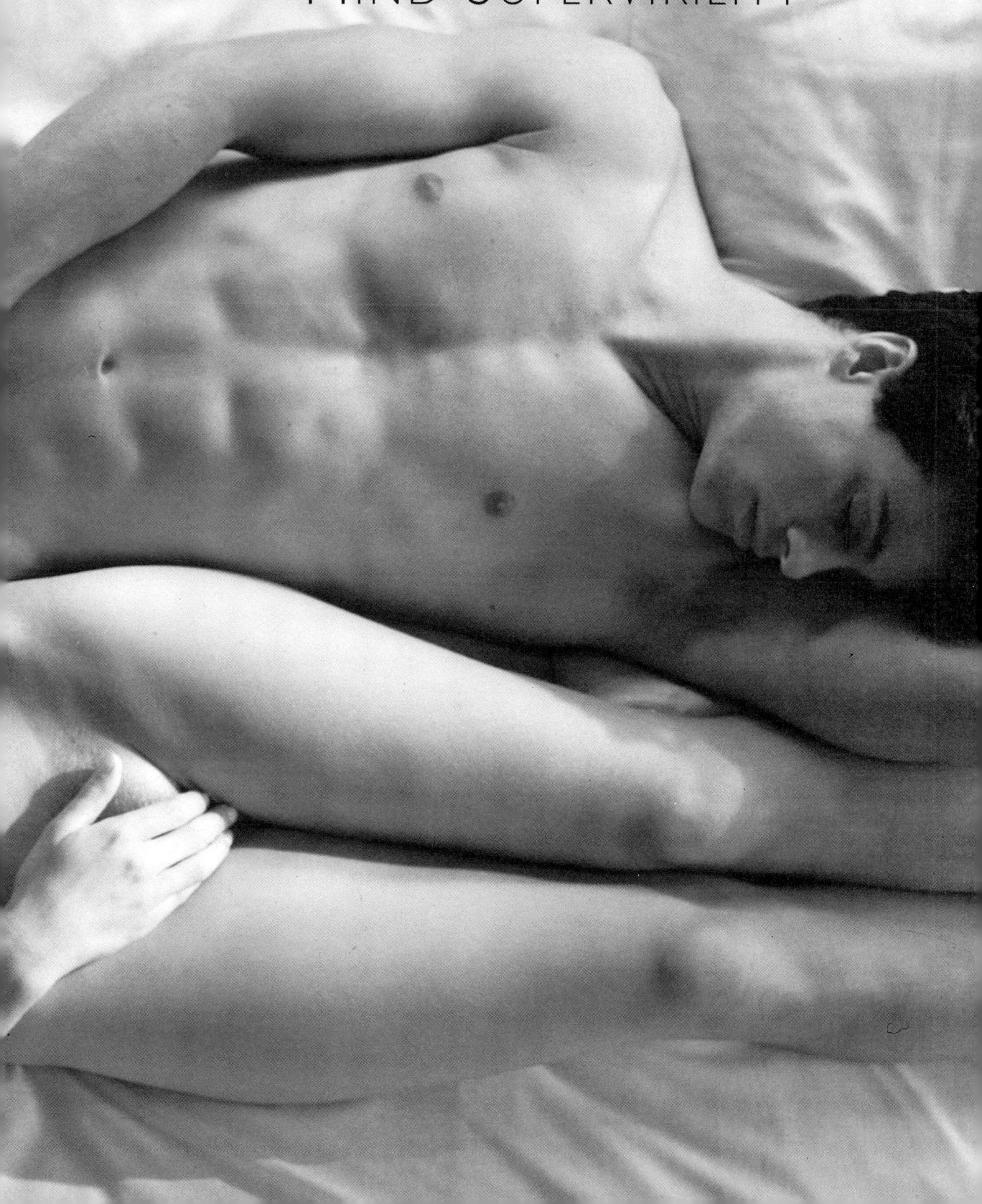

BREAKING FREE OF THE PAST

6

Don't think that only bodies determine sexual potential. Minds are just as important. For while your body provides the raw material for pleasure, it is your mind that controls just how much pleasure you feel, how much joy you take in being with a partner and how much sex means to you. In far too much love-making, it is your mind that blocks you off from Supervirility.

To understand why, you need to understand how minds work. We mentioned earlier that arousal is created when your brain responds to your five senses, and then sends messages of desire throughout your body. But overlaying this physical explanation is another, equally truthful psychological one – that it is what you *think* about what you see, hear and feel that creates arousal; it is the thoughts, feelings and fantasies you have that make you feel sexual by stimulating your brain. One thing is certainly true: the more powerful the picture, sound or word that is in your mind, the more powerfully it affects your brain, and the more powerful your arousal.

Not all these thoughts and feelings are in your conscious mind, however, which makes the whole process far more unpredictable. Consciously you may see something that turns you on, but subconsciously your mind may flinch, registering that now is not the time, that this is not the person, or that last time you were aroused you got emotionally hurt. You will withdraw from sex, but never realize why. So be aware that your mind may have some surprises in store for you, particularly around the issues of sexuality.

Past Influences

When we make love, it can seem as if we are living totally in the here and now. We can feel completely concentrated on what is happening in the present, to the exclusion of all else.

In fact, this is not what is happening at all. Although we don't realize it, everything that has happened in our life to date is affecting the way we make love. We bring into bed memories of thoughts, emotions and experiences that influence the way we react, feel and move in the present. Most of these messages are outside our consciousness; many of them were dropped into our minds many years ago, but they still affect us: limiting what we do and making us wary, or allowing us to be hopeful and building our confidence. They form what we might call our 'intimacy maps', our mental concepts of what love and sex mean, and who we are as a loving, sexual person.

Firstly, our information comes from our own direct experience of the sensations of sex. Whether we start at two with our hand down our knickers, or find at twelve that we can make 'it' go hard when we touch it, we will at some point in our lives begin to discover that there are wonderful things to be experienced through our own bodies.

But, conversely, other people will be giving us other messages. We may be told outright as children that intimate partnerships are wonderful (or wrong, or dangerous, or a waste of time). If we ourselves mention sex, or even worse do it – perhaps by touching or masturbating ourselves – then we also get a direct message from those around us, who support us or shout at us, give us more information or stop us from ever asking for information again. But most adults don't actually like being direct with children about sexuality or about intimacy. So, as we grow, we also get indirect messages. Perhaps we hear adults talking about sex, or see them reacting to a page three girl. Maybe we catch sight of a courting couple in a shop doorway, or overhear talk in the changing room. We not only pick up on what we see and hear, but also take on board other people's emotions about relationships – their pleasure, their outrage, their embarrassment, their lack of confidence. We don't only learn facts about sex, we also learn feelings.

Tracking Down the Messages

Learnings about sex come from all directions.

- **From our family and upbringing.** Our parents usually try to pass on their views about sex to us, in two ways. Firstly, they may well end up passing on a view simply because they are worried about our misusing sex in some way. However much people enjoy sex when they are growing up, there seems to be a built-in traditionalism that takes hold when they get children of their own, and become convinced that, in young hands, sex is a powerful and subversive tool! If this message is accompanied by positive messages about how enjoyable, as well as powerful, sex is, then we can often develop a very good attitude to sex. If not, we may end up feeling guilty.

  Or we may grow up in a family where sexual expression is encouraged – and this can be a problem, too. If a parent is overtly sexual to us, even in minor ways, before we can handle the enormous feelings involved, then we are in an emotional double-bind. We can't shrug off their actions, for it is a demand from an adult we depend on. We can't respond to it, for it may totally shatter our family and so remove the security we rely upon. In its worst manifestation, this is incest and leads to all kinds of self-blame and inhibition around sex; in its least harmful manifestation, we can still end up with the impression that sex is too powerful to handle, simply because we were exposed to it so early that we could not cope.

- **From culture and religion.** Many cultures and religions are confused about sex and unable to give young people working guidelines to help them cope in the real world. We may end up believing that sex is a sin, or that we have to love other people in order to be a good person, that men don't show their feelings, or that only a virgin is good enough to marry. If we do, then these beliefs, backed up by holy scripture and centuries of tradition, will stay with us for life and pop back up even when we think we have stopped believing them. Sound traditional beliefs, on the other hand, are those which stress the positivity of sex whilst also telling us how to cope with it and its dangers in everyday life.

- **From a single, one-off trauma.** In a recent survey run by a national group of magazines, one in ten men in Britain said they had been sexually harassed, and a horrifying one in twenty claimed to have been sexually assaulted, usually by other men. Sexual abuse, whether by family or strangers, whether as a child or an adult, is almost certain to create very strong feelings about sex and relationships. We may be wary of ever initiating sex or of ever enjoying it – and we may be nervous of ever forming intimate relationships, in case we get betrayed again. If we don't get emotional support to heal us, our desire may fade, never to re-emerge; our erection may fail and need much encouragement to rise in the future; we may hold back from ejaculating and find difficulty in ever doing so again.

- **From friends and peers.** We often get most of our sexual information from friends. Usually, this is based on disinformation and a need to seem better than anyone else. If, as boys reach adolescence, they feel a bit insecure, they can boost their ego by pretending to know everything about sex, or by boasting, ('I had three of them last night.' 'She couldn't keep her hands off me.') That sort of talk leaves everyone else feeling confused and slightly inferior.

- **From our general life relationships.** Every relationship we have during our life gives us ideas about love and hence about sex. Do we learn – from friends, relatives, colleagues and bosses – that people can be trusted, that we can expect people to stay with us, that it is who we are rather than what we do that matters? Or do we learn that people are going to run out on us, that we can't trust anyone, or that performance is everything? Is it any wonder, as we tumble into bed, that we hold back, keeping a masculine stiff upper lip and panicking if we don't 'perform' well? If we grow up with a sense of our own worth and a trust in other people, we will be far less anxious in bed, far more able to enjoy fully what is happening

- **From sexual partners.** Once we have bridged the gap into sexual relationships, the lessons multiply. And, because sex is so wonderful, and raises such strong sensations and emotions, the lessons are twice as crucial. Because we are never taught to make love, and at the same time taught to expect it will move mountains, we may learn confused lessons about sex or feel bad about it all. Alternatively, of course, over the years, sensitive and sensible lovers can provide us with a wealth of past experiences that allow us to enjoy and profit from our sexuality.

The Essential Contradiction

It becomes clear that most men end up with very mixed messages from the past about every aspect of what it means to be a sexual person. Studies show that all these messages can be classified into two distinct strands that underpin all our beliefs and all our attitudes.

First, we know from our own experience that sex is, on every physical level, quite wonderful. The sensations of arousal, of excitement, of erection and of orgasm all overwhelm us when we first experience them and continue to compel us back to repeat them, time and time again.

But, secondly, parallel to this, many messages we receive from those around us tell us that sex can be bad, wrong, embarrassing or harmful. Perhaps because of religion or perhaps because of fear, maybe because they know that it is a strong force, and maybe because they are wary of too much pleasure, generation after generation of human beings persist in passing on the myth that really, at bottom, sex is wrong. The deduction we obviously draw from this is that, if we long for sex, then we ourselves are wrong. We begin to doubt ourselves, our masculinity, our sexuality.

So we struggle with the essential contradiction. Sex is good and yet it is bad. We want it and yet we are wrong to want it. We are attracted to it then pull away from it. Our minds, stimulated by arousal, are also stimulated by anxiety – we go towards sex, but we also withdraw.

And, when we come face to face with with sex itself, as we initiate it, move into arousal, get an erection or reach orgasm, we constantly trigger these contradictions. Present sexuality is a hotline into past events, with positive and negative emotions flooding through.

Where Are You Now?

Now check your own attitudes against those listed here, and start to track just where you need to break free of the past.

- **Shutting down desire.** Perhaps things have happened in our early lives to make us angry or fearful about sex, or anxious about ourselves as sexual men – our parents' anger, our religious leaders' warnings. The double-bind pull between pleasure and guilt leaves us anxious; even if we are unaware of it, we may be wary of ever feeling aroused. At the very point that we begin to do so, we automatically shut off our desire. Though the newness of our current partnership overrode this, once that became stable, this pattern re-established itself. Slowly, over the years, this shut-off backs up, and we now shut off earlier and earlier as we feel aroused. In the end, we only feel sexual when an override happens, a sudden rush of physical feeling triggered by erotica; a lowering of inhibitions when we get drunk; a coming together in crisis or in celebration. Otherwise, we have lost our desire.

  Or, because of things that have happened in our early lives to make us relaxed and confident about sex and about our masculinity, we welcome arousal when it comes. Despite any experiences to the contrary, we maintain desire throughout our lives.

- **Stepping back from the feelings.** Maybe we learn that emotions are problematic. When tempted to feel any of the 'soft' emotions, such as sadness, compassion, fear, affection, enthusiasm, embarrassment, or guilt, we shut down on these and refuse to experience them. We become unable to feel emotion, or to link it with sexual experience in any way. We maybe do this even to the point

SUPERVIRILITY

where we mentally step outside our bodies when we make love, and 'spectate' on what we are doing as if we were mere observers – so our love-making becomes mechanical and fraught.

Or, we learn to feel a full range of emotions, including the 'soft' ones, particularly when we are making love, and so are able to enter fully into the experience of sexuality with mind as well as body.

- **Getting bored with sex.** We learn from the past that it is not acceptable to ask for what we want, so we stick with our usual patterns of sex, and never initiate any new ones. We remember our mother's disapproving face when we asked for something as a child, and we feel wary. We think of pointing out when some part of sex is not enjoyable, and feel the same negative feeling. We stick to the safety of what we know. And, ultimately, inevitably, sex loses its charm, and we feel bored.

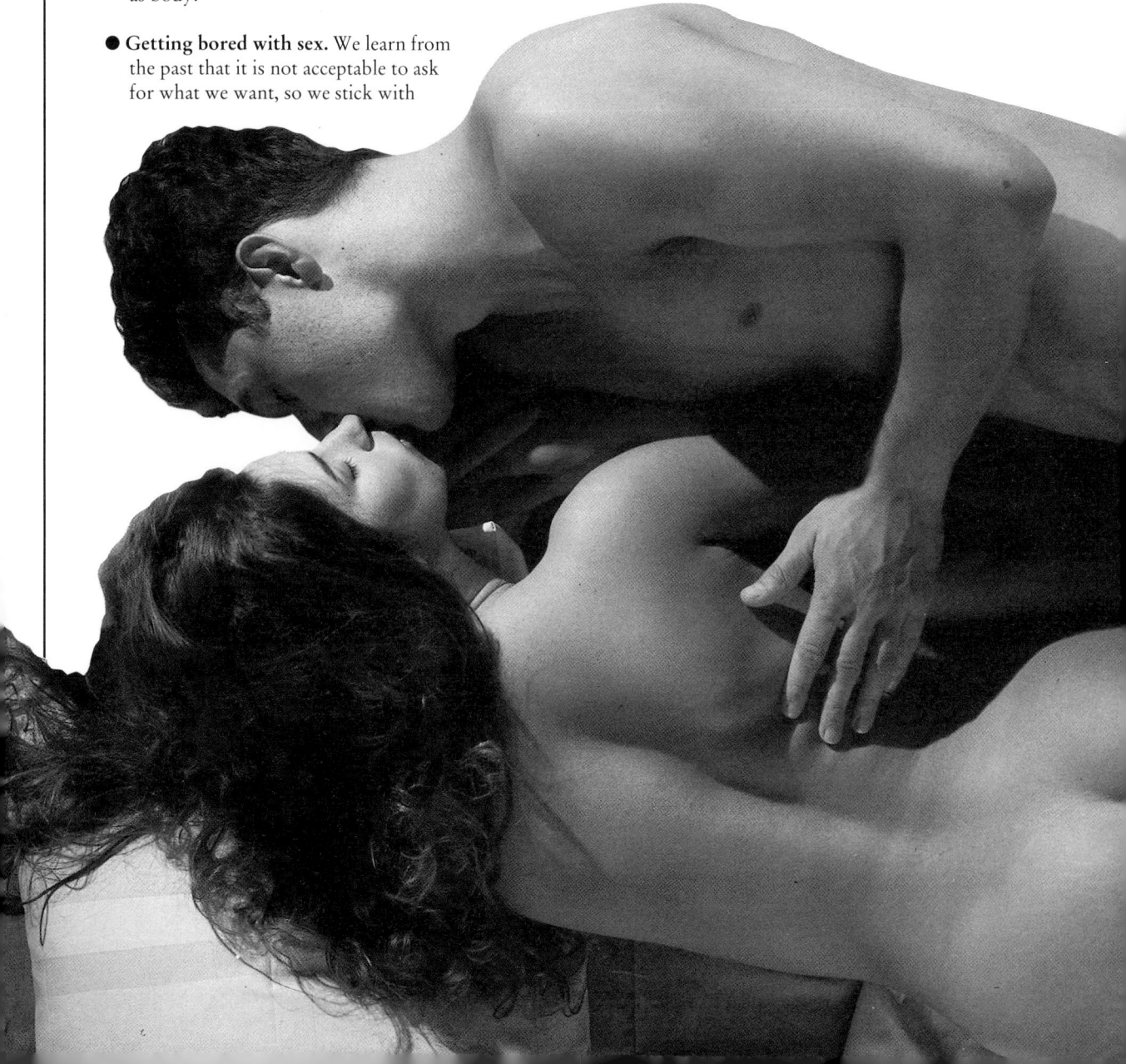

Breaking Free of the Past

Or, we are confident about suggesting new things or requesting that unenjoyable sex be changed – not because we know we will always get what we want, but because we have memories of being accepted as a child when we asked for things. We are able to adapt our sex life to one that always meets our needs and that of our partner – so avoiding boredom.

- **Going into a failure spiral.** Past events, possibly traumatic ones, seeded the fear that we wouldn't be able to succeed in things. A trigger incident in the present puts the thought into our minds, maybe with particular reference to erection or ejaculation. We run that thought round and round our heads, becoming more and more panicked as we do so. Next time, fearfully and possibly guiltily, we try. Our anxiety itself sabotages our good intentions; we are proved right when we fail to get an erection. Our fear grows, creating even more of a self-fulfilling prophecy for next time.

  Or, past events have made us confident that even if something goes wrong, we will be able to overcome it in time. So if we can't get it up at some point, we relax and dismiss the problem from our mind. Very soon, with no anxiety to stop it, our sexuality returns of its own accord.

- **Feeling sex is dirty.** We have learned all too well the lesson that sex is dirty or bad, maybe from parents or teachers who were themselves disgusted with sex or thought it was immoral. At the back of our minds, maybe out of our consciousness, we are uneasy with the physical aspects of sex, we think of the possibility that our partner may get pregnant, or have the feeling that our partner is too good to soil by having sex with her. We shut off in our minds the sheer pleasure and fulfilment of sex, and so fight shy of ejaculation and find it difficult to reach orgasm.

Or, our early messages were about sex being natural and normal; the suggestion that it is dirty would make no sense to us. So we are able to make love with our minds focusing entirely on the pleasure.

- **Being afraid of pleasure.** We have a deep-rooted belief that we are so bad that we don't really deserve pleasure in sex. Alternatively, we have learned from sad experience, maybe with an angry father who caught us masturbating, or a displeased girlfriend who wanted all the attention on her, that if we do allow ourselves pleasure, something awful will happen. We come very quickly, to get the pleasure over with – or find it extremely difficult to come, in order to delay the inevitable punishment.

    Or, we know that pleasure sometimes has its problems, but we also know that we don't need to feel guilty or punished if we enjoy ourselves. We are happy to come when we do, able to hang on longer if we wish to, or go for a quickie if that is what we want.

- **Getting totally paralysed.** An early trauma or a very strict upbringing may leave a very small minority of us unable to have any sexual response at all. Primary sexual blocks – never having been able to have an erection or to ejaculate – are occasionally caused this way, and need specialist counselling.

Be reassured, by the way, that everyone suffers from some of the blocks we describe; no one is totally together about sex!

WHEN THE PAST HOOKS YOU

It is possible to break down the blocks, even the ones that come from the very distant past, so that they lose their hold on you. You have taken the first step in doing so just by reading this chapter, for in recognizing that some of your attitudes come from past events – and by realizing that these attitudes dictate your sexuality – you are several leaps ahead of many people.

The next move is to recognize that, if while in bed you hit a block that comes from the distant past, you can't expect just to charge on through and ignore it. You may mentally berate yourself for having such stupid thoughts, or cursing yourself for having that particular memory at such an inappropriate time. Don't. By hitting yourself over the head, you are just adding to the problem. Instead, stop love-making and cuddle; hold your partner close, use some of the relaxation or deep-breathing techniques we mention in Chapter 2 – and congratulate yourself.

For by bringing to your attention this particular thought or this particular memory, your mind is doing you a favour; it is jumping up and down to point out that this event from your past is holding you back from Supervirility. So take the time, either in bed or later, to think through the mental link you made. If you are close to your partner, tell her about your memory, and explore together how it is stopping you doing what you want in bed.

Even if you have no direct memories brought to your attention by love-making, you will already have some inkling of how the past affects you, just by reading through the examples we have included in this chapter. If you shivered when you read about being caught masturbating, or flinched at the section on religion, then these are areas of vulnerability for you.

BREAKING FREE

And you can be more precise in tracking these areas down. Begin by taking a quiet half an hour with pen and paper.

1. First, think about yourself in the present day, as a sexual man, in your situation, at this particular time.

2. Then, look at the chart on page 62. We have listed out some key people who may have given you messages about sexuality, your identity as a sexual man, and intimate relationships. If we have missed out any particular people who are significant in your life, then add them in.

3. For each person or group of people, identify and write down one message. Did your mother tell you not to get anyone pregnant? Did your best friend make it clear that you weren't getting it as much as he was? What messages have important people in your life given you? Add in, too, any particular memories that love-making has raised for you.

4. Remember that these messages may have been given to you on just one occasion: your parents finding you masturbating in the bathroom; or over a long period of time: a series of girlfriends who wouldn't sleep with you. As you write in each key message, start becoming aware of whether you took it in instantly, on one occasion, or slowly over time.

5. Also, remember that the messages you got may not have been overtly about sex – having a friend in school who let you down may now mean that you have less trust in every relationship, including intimate ones. So trawl back not only over sexual memories but also over any others that have influenced you.

6. When you've completed your list, go back to each message in turn. Ask yourself these questions about it.

- How is this message affecting me here and now?

- Has it given me a positive belief in what sex means and how good it is, in who I am and how sexual I am?

- Or does the message carry a negative connotation, that makes me feel less good about sex and about myself?

- How do these messages affect what I do in bed and how I do it? Are these messages creating any blocks for me sexually at the moment?

What positive messages have you noted down? Begin to reinforce them. Simple mental strategies often work best. Write out a positive belief you feel good about; carry it around in your wallet or pop it in a bedside drawer. Every time you catch sight of it, allow yourself to smile at the fact that your sexuality is enhanced by your positive belief.

At the start of each day, maybe when you are cleaning your teeth, take a moment to look back over the preceding twenty-four hours and realize how your positive belief about yourself has influenced you. Maybe the fact that you learned early in life that touching was OK allowed you to give your partner a hug last night when she needed it – or to snuggle up to her and initiate sex this morning. Once you begin to become aware of how your past is positively influencing your present, you will start to build confidence that you can make your entire past work for you.

When you have identified negative messages from the past, you can begin to take a new perspective on them. Firstly, make sure that you are clear just how non-useful they are, just how much they are stopping you from fulfilling your sexual potential.

SUPERVIRILITY

Key People	Messages
Mother	
Father	
Religious leaders	
Brothers or sisters	
Friends	
Colleagues	
Sexual partners	
Present sexual partner	

Next, put your negative messages to the test. Get facts about whether masturbation really makes you go blind, as your brother once told you; discuss your feelings about oral sex with your partner.

With this new information, think back to the event or events where you learned the messages you carry and begin to rethink them. Ask yourself these questions:

● What was really going on when I was given that message? Looking at what was happening from the outside, what were the other people really feeling and doing? (Your dad shouted at you not because you were bad but because he felt threatened... your girlfriends said no to you not because they didn't like you but because they were frightened of sex.)

● Now, looking back on it from an adult perspective, what do I realize about what happened that I never realized before? (That masturbation isn't a sin... that, in the end, you would find a loving relationship.)

● What could I have realized that would have given me a much more positive and useful message about sex and about myself as a sexual person? (That it's OK to give myself pleasure... that I am a lovable person.)

You'll find, if you keep stepping back in time like this to take a new perspective and realize what you didn't learn previously, that, in the end, your negative messages will fade away.

However, in order finally to break free of the past, you may need to recognize that you can't do it alone. If one of your early memories is a very traumatic one, such as incest, then you may need outside help to come to terms with it. There is no reason why it should continue to mess up your life, and we would strongly recommend that you use Appendix A to find a counsellor who can help you.

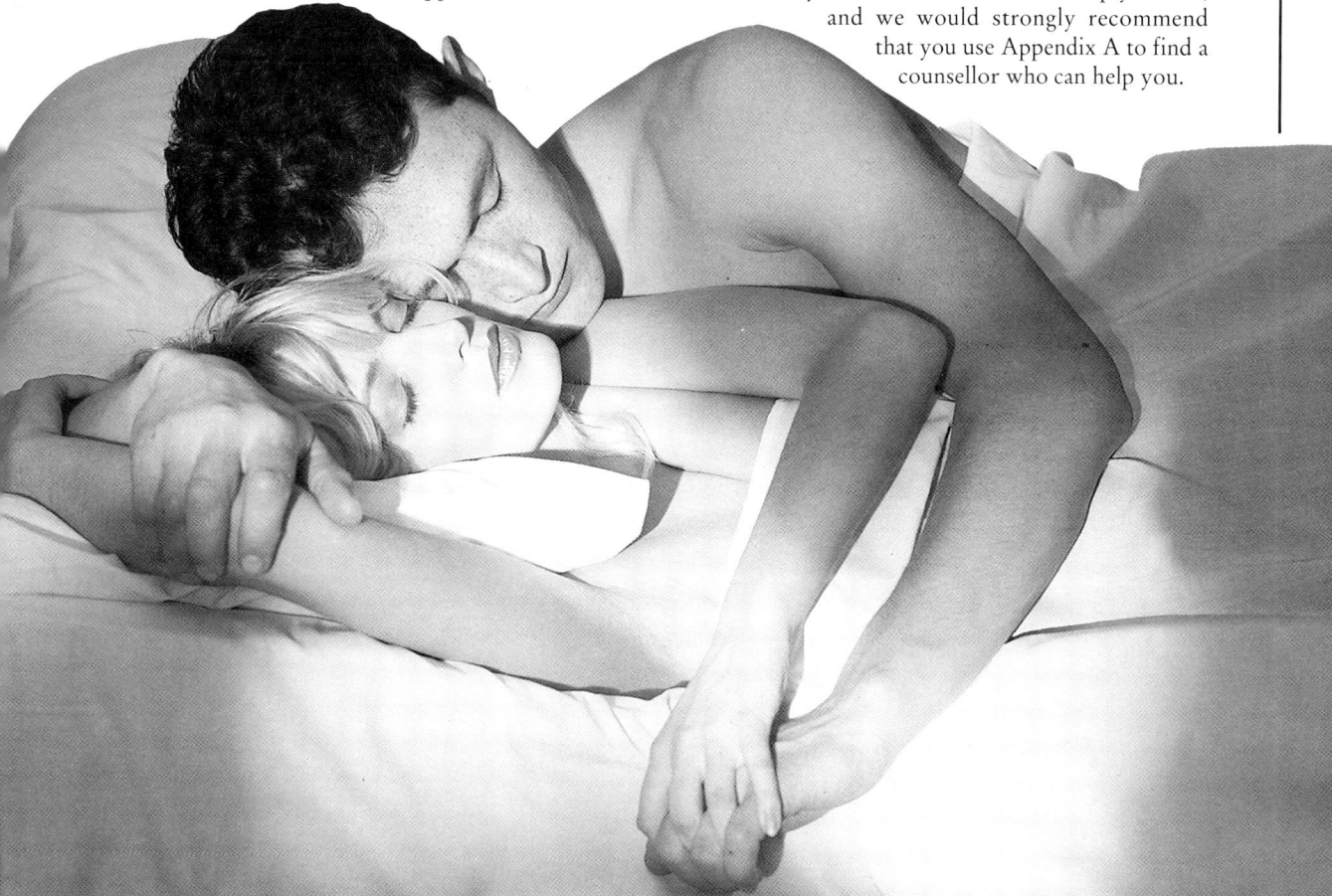

7 Sexual Myths

We are surrounded by myths about sex. A real man gets it up all the time. A real woman wants it all the time. Real sex is about doing it all the time. And every time we hear a myth and mentally believe it, our minds become less and less able to create a good sex life for our bodies.

Where do we get these messages from? The media promote a vision of myth-based sex because they think that's what people want. Men themselves often perpetuate the myths because they are afraid that challenging them may make other men, who do buy into it, think they are inferior. And then perhaps they mask fears by exaggerating their own performance in conversation with friends and so pass the myth on down the line to the young men who come after.

Read this sample list of myths that every man is asked to reckon with. You may not believe all of them, may not even consider that you believe any of them – but think carefully, as you read the list, about how many of them lurk at the corner of your mind, digging away at your – or your partner's – self-esteem even now.

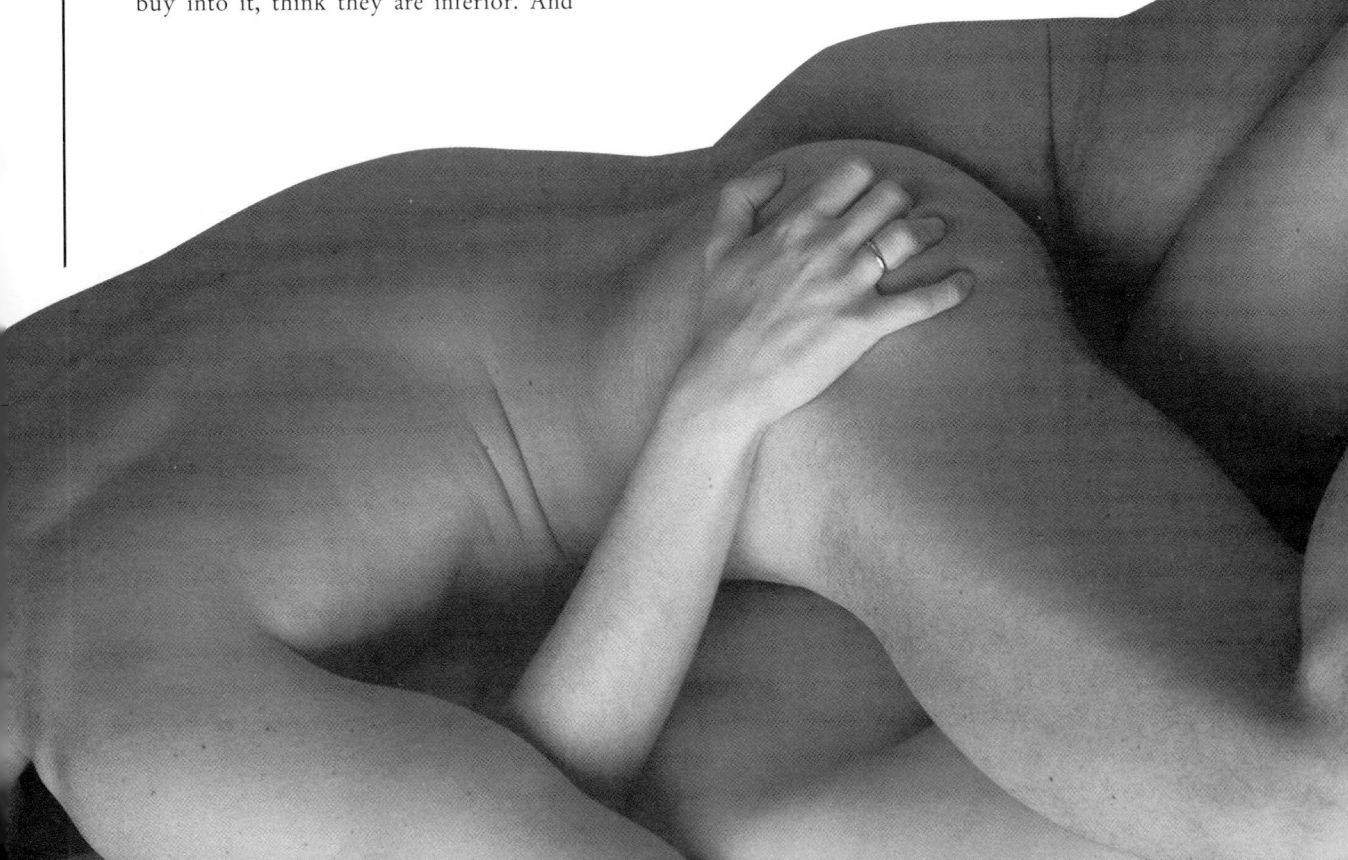

Sexual Myths

The Myths

A real man...
- has a big penis;
- is always hard;
- is always ready for it;
- must be active;
- knows what to do without being told;
- must be responsible for his partner's pleasure;
- will naturally give his partner multiple orgasms; and
- mustn't feel or show his feelings.

A real woman...
- is always ready for sex;
- is aroused quickly;
- loves big penises;
- love penetration; and
- does what you want in bed all the time.

Real sex...
- is down to performance;
- needs an erection;
- means intercourse;
- always leads to orgasm, preferably simultaneous.

Now let's go through the list again debunking the myths.

A real man...

- **has a big penis.** Let us repeat that most penises are about the same size when erect. When you make love, your partner's vagina expands or contracts to accommodate the penis available, and so it doesn't matter how big or small it is. What matters is how you use it.

- **is always hard.** Very young men often walk around with a hard-on for days. Once you're getting it regularly, this is no longer so imperative, and most men respond only when appropriate. In any case, for most women, a hard penis is not what love-making is about.

- **is always ready for it.** Actually, no. Most men who have a full life involving partner, family and career like regular sex, but want the freedom to be in the mood rather than doing it on demand.

- **must be active.** Many men love being passive and letting their partner take over. Many women love that, too.

- **knows what to do without being told.** Would you try to play the concert violin without training? Doing what comes naturally is one thing, but if you take sex seriously, you should be prepared to learn.

- **must be responsible for his partner's pleasure.** This seems very hard on the man. Mutual responsibility seems to us to be what sex and relationships are about.

- **will give his partner multiple orgasms.** It is nice to work together to give you both as many orgasms as you want – but remember that, for many women, one orgasm is a victory.

- **mustn't feel or show his feelings.** Good sex is enhanced by exchanging emotional expression during sex as well as before and after it. Men who buy into this myth become emotional 'withholders', cutting themselves off from a key source of sensation and pleasure – as well as, in the long run, cutting themselves off from their partners.

SUPERVIRILITY

A REAL WOMAN...

- **is always ready for sex.** Like men, women have times when they want sex and times when they don't.

- **is aroused quickly.** The female anatomy often lends itself to a slow build-up to sex, and many women get aroused more slowly than men. Both men and women should have the option for long, slow love-making or quickies, depending on the mood.

- **loves big penises.** In numerous studies, women asked what they most liked about men didn't mention penis size at all. Obviously some women do judge on quantity, but in general it is not nearly so important to them as the quality of how a penis is used.

- **loves penetration.** Many women love the feeling of being penetrated by the man they love. But, as we explain later in the book, female biology means that penetration often fails to touch the parts that are important, so many women get no actual physical pleasure from standard intercourse.

- **does what you want in bed all the time.** Some women do concentrate on only pleasing their man and ignore pleasure for themselves but, if they do, in the long run their bodies rebel and they get turned off sex altogether. Both sexes ignore this warning at their peril.

REAL SEX...

- **is down to performance.** If we as authors could expunge any myth from the face of the earth, it would be this one. For too many men, sex is about performance; if men were allowed to relax and see sex as something playful and relaxed, male sexual effectiveness would rise by one thousand per cent.

- **needs an erection.** There are many wonderful ways to have sex with your partner without your having an erection at all. The pleasure you can have from love-making all over your body can be at least equal to the pleasure you can have from an erection.

- **means intercourse.** See our comments above about the mixed blessings of penetration. Many people get better and stronger orgasms from mouth or hand sex than from intercourse.

- **always leads to orgasms, preferably simultaneous.** It is nice if orgasms happen eventually – but the pleasure of keeping going in the pre-orgasmic plateau phase is also good. Simultaneous orgasms are fun, but not nearly as common as some sex manuals would have you believe.

Surely myths are a problem on several levels. Firstly, they give us disinformation, leading us to believe things that simply aren't true; when we believe them, we end up undermining love-making simply because we aren't getting the right information to start with. Secondly, particular myths can underpin particular problems, and that can hold you back from Supervirility. For all these myths have a hidden imperative in them, a 'should' that tells you what you really ought to be, and the way you really ought to perform. Your mind, very sensibly, reacts to all the myths that include a 'should' by digging its heels in, like any small boy, and saying 'won't'.

Try to remember that:

- Any of the myths that stress how wonderful real men are, or how incredible real sex is, can undermine your desire, convincing you that, because you don't match up to the ideal, you don't deserve to have sex. This will make you anxious every time you even think of it, and so ultimately make the whole thing not worth the bother.

- The same mechanism operates with erectile dysfunction. It only takes a slight diminishing of your erection for you to start comparing yourself with the mythical Wonderman – and panicking. Panic is the foundation of all too many erectile problems, as your mind cowers in a corner and refuses to raise the flag.

- The whole gamut of myths around staying in control and being unemotional affects the ability to let go sufficiently to come. So believing any of the myths about real men doing it all on their own are going to make you less able to really enjoy your orgasm – or even unable to have one at all. The same goes for any myth about having to have an orgasm.

- And, of course, all the myths about real women set up horrendous barriers between you and your partner, barriers that will bar you from being a truly intimate and loving couple who are capable of an incredible sex life.

DEBUNKING THE MYTHS

The first thing you can do to debunk the myths is to get rightfully angry. These myths are a con trick, which puts pressure on men and makes them perform to order. At the same time they do not allow them the real resources they need to make sex successful. Perhaps no one is to blame for these myths – which began in the mists of time – but that is no reason why men shouldn't be angry about them and their effects.

Longer term, there is practical action you can take to debunk the myths in your own mind. Choose a myth – any myth – that you have previously bought into. Call on all your knowledge of yourself and your partner to back up your suspicion that this myth is wrong. Talk to your partner about it and discuss her feelings. Read any of the current books on men's feelings, such as the *Hite Report on Male Sexuality*.

Then think how you could most contradict the myth you've been taken in by. By being totally passive in bed during the next three love-making sessions? By only going for oral sex for the next month? If you find that a particular myth steals into your consciousness in bed – so that you give yourself a hard time because you aren't a stud, or feel guilty because you are showing your emotion – remember that you are being conned. Stop and have a good laugh about it, then play-act the worst sex you can possibly imagine. That should lighten you both up for next time!

There is something else you can do, too. Teach others. It may be too scary to challenge the myths when you hear them bandied about in the changing room after football. But you could, when telling your son or daughter about sex, make it clear that the myths are not descriptions of real people making real love. Maybe if everyone taught this to the next generation then a good proportion of all sexual hang-ups would disappear overnight.

COPING WITH STRESS

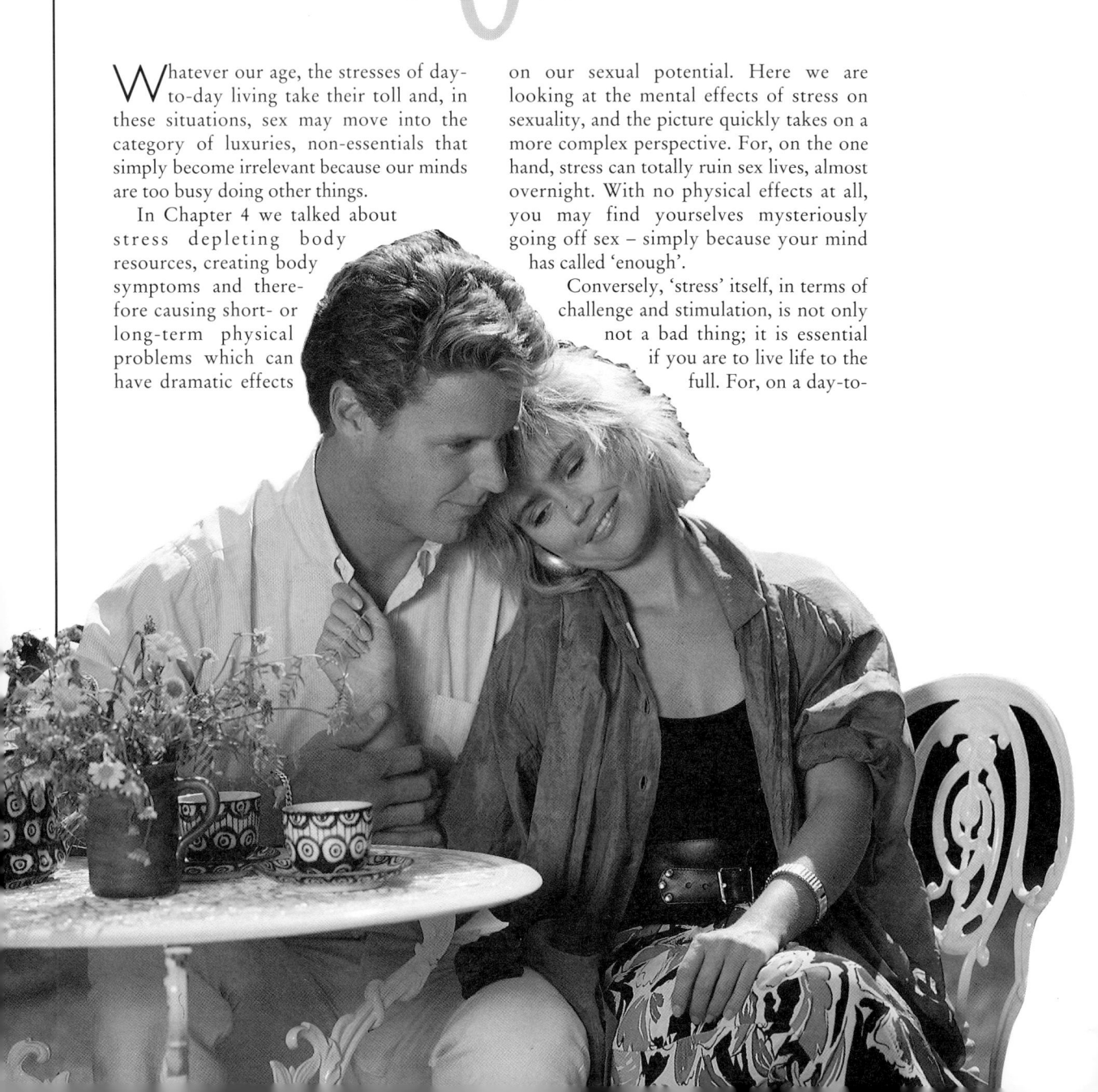

8

Whatever our age, the stresses of day-to-day living take their toll and, in these situations, sex may move into the category of luxuries, non-essentials that simply become irrelevant because our minds are too busy doing other things.

In Chapter 4 we talked about stress depleting body resources, creating body symptoms and therefore causing short- or long-term physical problems which can have dramatic effects on our sexual potential. Here we are looking at the mental effects of stress on sexuality, and the picture quickly takes on a more complex perspective. For, on the one hand, stress can totally ruin sex lives, almost overnight. With no physical effects at all, you may find yourselves mysteriously going off sex – simply because your mind has called 'enough'.

Conversely, 'stress' itself, in terms of challenge and stimulation, is not only not a bad thing; it is essential if you are to live life to the full. For, on a day-to-day level, everyone needs some kind of challenging occurrence to keep them psychologically alert, confident in themselves and sexually active. In the long run, a totally unchallenging existence makes people lose confidence, begin to see themselves negatively and, as a result, sexual performance quickly nose-dives. Supervirility is not just a case of leading a quiet life.

FINDING THE BALANCE

The answer to getting the balance right lies in the mind: for it is how people react to life's events on a mental level that determines whether they get overwhelmed by them, that determines whether the physical horrors we described in Chapter 4 come into play. If, in your mind, you cope with what is happening around you, then you can walk the thin dividing line that exists between too much stimulation and too little, and your sex life will remain active and successful.

To understand this mechanism, first look briefly at six life events that can affect us:

- Bereavement;
- Promotion;
- Moving house;
- Family celebration;
- Meeting a work deadline; and
- Redundancy.

Some of these are obviously mentally undermining. Bereavement will take its toll on anyone. Others may seem to be positive occasions but also contain the germs of stress – in the extra responsibility of promotion, for example, or the hassle of moving house. For the stress factor of success is equal to that of failure – and, often, the support available is far less. Equally, elements which seem totally negative have positive sides to them. If a redundancy is approached with fear it may well deflate erection for months to come, while if it is the opportunity of a lifetime to start a new company and leave a boring job, redundancy can raise sex life to a peak not achieved in years.

To create a sex life that is not undermined by stress, you need to keep balanced in terms of stimulation. You need to look at what is happening in your life, and make sure that you have:

- some situations or events that allow you mentally and emotionally to relax and let go;

- some situations or events that stimulate and challenge, so that mentally you feel proud of yourself;

- a minimum number of situations and events that seem so negative that they put you under unrelieved stress;

- an ability to respond to obviously 'negative' situations or events with a positive attitude, to make sure that they don't overwhelm you and mentally sap your confidence; and

- the ability to get support in situations in which it is obviously difficult to have a positive attitude.

How does this relate to your life, and in particular to any sexual blocks you may be hitting? It is difficult without an in-depth exploration to link a particular area of sexual dissatisfaction with the balance of stress in your life and how you are coping with it; in terms of this book, we simply don't know your situation well enough.

We can however, offer you a way to ascertain in general whether mental stress is threatening your sex life.

Assessing Your Stress Level

Beside the following list of potentially stressful life elements, only mark the ones that are happening to you at present. If you find that a particular event or situation is **relaxing** for you, tick the **R** box. If you find a situation or event actually **challenging** and **stimulating**, despite its potentially stressful elements, then tick the **C** box. If you find the situation totally **negative**, and it is overwhelming you, then tick the **N** box. If you know that the element is potentially stressful, but you feel you are successfully looking on the **positive** side, then tick the **P** box. If you are getting sufficient **support** to handle it, then instead tick the **S** box.

Situations	R	C	N	P	S
Child(ren) leave(s) home					
Child(ren) leave(s) school					
Christmas					
Conviction for an offence					
Cooking					
Day off					
Day out					
Death of friend					
Death of partner					
Different work responsibilities					
Direct relaxation					
Divorce					
Do It Yourself					
Driving					
Early retirement					
Evening out with family					
Evening in with family					
Exercise class					
Family bereavement					
Gardening					
Giving up smoking					
Going on holiday					
Going out for a meal					
Going shopping for food					
Going shopping for personal items					
House repossession					
Housework					
Illness					
Illness of close family					
In-law problems					
Injury					
Injury of close family					
Job change					
Listening to music					
Loan shopping					

Coping with Stress

Situations	R	C	N	P	S
Loss of job					
Lowered work load					
Marriage					
Massage					
Meeting a deadline at work					
Money worries					
Mortgage					
Moving house					
New child					
New job					
New project at work					
Passed over for promotion					
Pay cut					
Pay rise					
Playing important sports match					
Playing sport					
Playing with children					
Promotion					
Raised work load					
Redecorating at home					
Retirement					
Separation					
Significant birthday (e.g., 30, 40, 50)					
Starting new eating patterns					
Taking up new sport					
Taking on a loan					
Taking a bath					
Taking a sauna					
Time in jail					
Visiting relatives					
Visiting friends					
Weekend					
Wife (re)starts work					
Work success					

Now look at the pattern you have created for yourself. If you have less than four **R**s, then you are not creating sufficient opportunity for yourself to let go and relax. Make sure you raise your **R** rating immediately.

If you have less than four **C**s, and no other marks on your sheet, then perhaps you are not stretching yourself enough. Don't try to create problems for yourself, but do look at ways in which you can take on more: more job responsibility, a further commitment, a work, relationship or leisure challenge.

More than four **N**s means that you are under sufficient strain that it may be affecting your sex life. Get extra support, from family, friends, professional therapists or counselling staff at work.

If you have six or more **P**s, then you obviously have an effective mental approach to life's challenges, although if that number rises, you may find that your tolerance and energy starts to slip and that you are unable to keep up your positive attitude.

If you have ticked more than four **S**s, then despite the fact that you are getting support, you are under too much strain for your sex life to be unaffected.

Taking Action

If a stress-producer in your life is short term, create a good family support system for yourself and get the situation sorted out. Avoid any kind of extra strain; don't, for example, start counselling or even take a major holiday while the situation is still going on. Expect some kick-backs even after problems are over, and make sure you have a mental and physical 'convalescence' period before you expect your sex life to return to normal.

If the situation threatens to become long term, then take a long-term view: build up physical health and make sure that you are relaxing mentally, too. Learn how to say no to people, so that you are not leant on in turn. Develop your time management skills and don't be afraid to ask people to do things for you in order to conserve your own energy. Take up a class or course in mental relaxation: meditation does not need to be linked to a particular philosophy and its simple mental exercises can calm you, allowing you to avoid the mental loops that create sexual failure. Autogenic training is similar to meditation but thoroughly Westernized in its approach – and claims in particular to have beneficial effects on stress-induced erectile problems.

In particular, if the stress you are under overwhelms you, and you move into depression, seek professional help immediately; depression can erase your sex life as if it had never existed – and, worse, create in you a mental apathy. This can leave you unconcerned whether your sexuality will ever reappear!

What if the issues you ticked cluster together in what might be called a midlife crisis, where you receive reminders of the passage of time? A significant birthday, being passed over for promotion, your partner taking a job, children leaving home – all these are intimations of mortality, and may leave you feeling down and powerless. They may make you frightened (by the future) and angry (at the irretrievable past), and they then show in your sexuality, bringing lack of confidence, loss of desire or erection failure in their wake.

If this is so, then you may need to change totally the way you see yourself and your life. You need to make a conscious effort to remind yourself of the good things – about being older, having a more secure relationship, more time to be relaxed and innovative about sex – and about how, in particular, some of your sexual blocks may actually ease as you age and become less dependent on urgent sexual release. To paraphrase Maurice Chevalier: 'The only difference between a man of twenty and a man of fifty is thirty years' experience!' Midlife, viewed from the correct perspective, means that you have everything going for you.

Your stress-created issue may, however, be much more specific than this. How can you cope with mental strain whilst actually making love, when the current stress-producer rushes into your mind, driving away desire or lowering your erection? Simply, stop immediately and take the pressure off yourself by cuddling and relaxing as fully as you can. As we have mentioned before, don't mentally scold yourself, which will only make you feel worse about your 'failure'; but neither let your mind draw you into further worrying about whatever crisis is upsetting you. Don't push forward to intercourse, but fall back to romance, kind words and courting behaviour again. If necessary, while you are under strain, don't even attempt sex for a few weeks, or you will turn it into just something else to worry about. If when you resume again because desire has risen, your confidence in your erection returning has suffered a knock, then use the explorations in Chapter 9 to restore your self-belief and get back on top again.

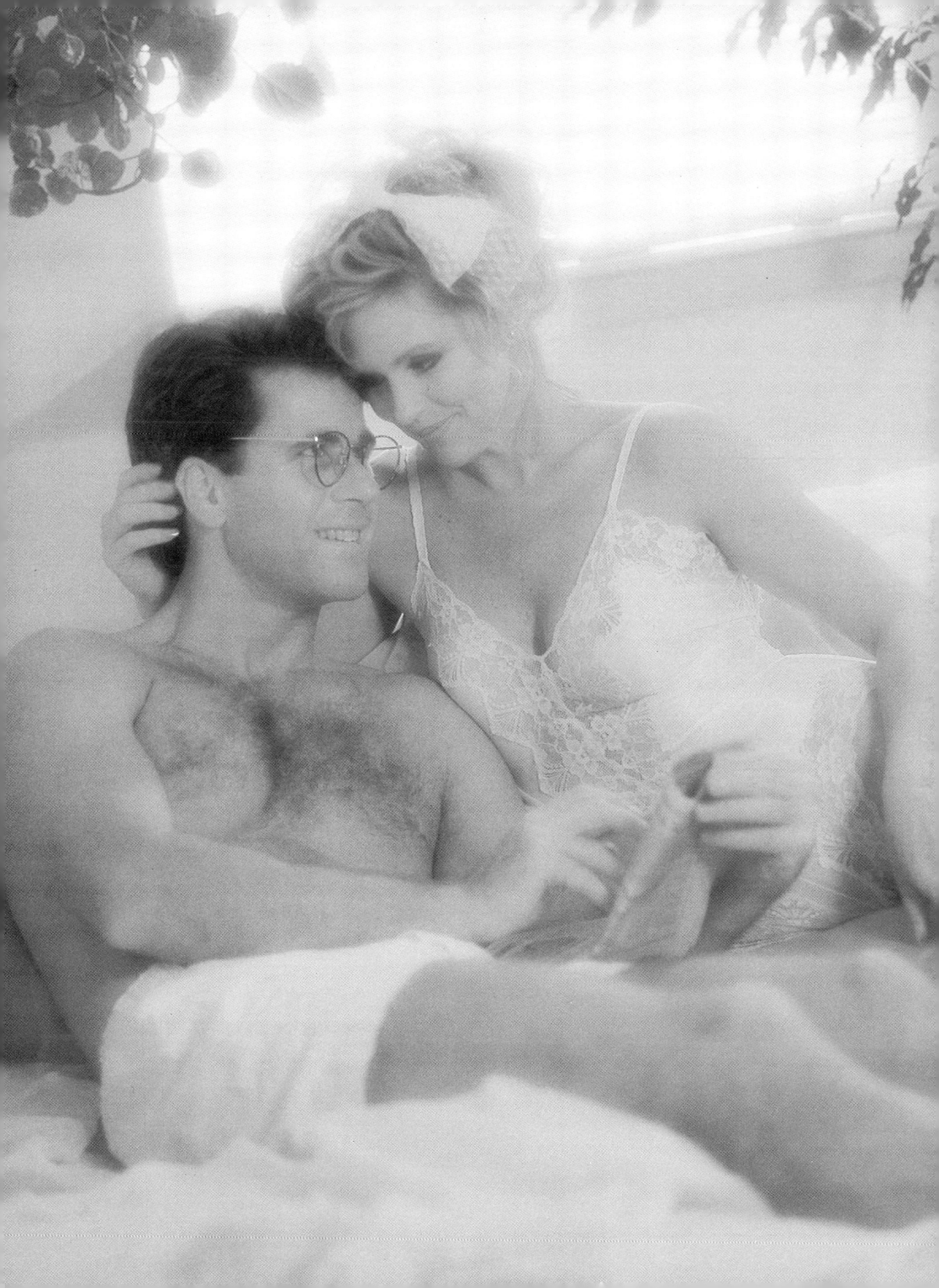

Building a Supervirile Personality

Time after time, women report that what makes a man a good lover is what he thinks, feels and says in bed rather than the size of his penis or his ability to last a long time.

So are we saying that you have to have a particular mental approach in order to have true Supervirility? Yes, we are. For it is, fundamentally, your personality showing through in sex that makes you Supervirile. Do you make sex fun? Are you confident about it? Are you able to accept as well as give pleasure? All the erotic positions in the world cannot compensate if you are tight-lipped, nervous and goal-oriented in bed. Conversely, if you are relaxed, self-confident and willing to let go, then you will sidestep any potential sexual blocks as if they never existed.

We asked a number of women we know just what attributes of a man's personality made sex a good experience for them. These are some of the answers we received:

'He feels really good about himself in bed.'

'He is fine about being asked to do something, or not to do something, in bed'...

'He feels he can ask for what he wants.'

'He is at ease with closeness and intimacy'

'Lots of emotion, whatever he feels...'

'He lets go when he's aroused, doesn't hang on to control all the time.'

'He's not fazed if it doesn't work occasionally.'

'No hang-ups, does anything, shares fantasies, tries different things.'

'He's really over the moon when things go well.'

We're not talking here about a façade of action. It isn't enough to pretend to be open-minded, or to act unworried about problems. The mind-set needs to go further than that, which is why you probably need to take action aimed at changing your approach on a deeper level.

We list the mental approaches you need one by one, explaining just what they involve and how you can develop them in yourself. Choose one at a time, then do the relevant exploration included in each. They are not all concerned with what you do in bed; some involve lead-up practice outside the bedroom. They are all, however, carefully planned so that you get the attitudes you need through the actions we suggest. Some of the explorations will prove easy, and within days you will have changed your approach. Others may take longer, and be more of a challenge. Some are actually quite daring and you may decide to leave them out. If so, that's fine.

Building a Supervirile Personality

'He feels really good about himself in bed.'

This essential personality trait underpins all the others needed for Supervirility. If you feel bad about yourself in bed, you risk a whole range of blocks: loss of desire, a fear of erection, an inability to come when you want. If you are able to feel good about yourself in bed, then you will give and receive good sex, with desire that lasts for ever and no problems. We are not talking here about being over-confident or, if you will pardon the pun, being cocky; it is about being sufficiently sure of yourself that anything that happens in bed – from total disaster to overwhelming success – leaves you and your partner secure and confident in yourselves. You are secure in your masculinity, whether or not you 'perform', and you are yourself in bed, warts and all. Such self-esteem makes you a fully sexual person.

Action: Take time to make a list of all the things you feel proud of in your life. If possible get other people (partner, kids, friends) to help. You will need to listen carefully if they congratulate you; otherwise, sheer embarrassment will block your hearing! Your list might include having a good sense of humour, building the extension, caring for your partner when your first baby was born, cooking a great meal. When you've completed the list, bask in what you've done – and add to it regularly. This is probably one of the most challenging explorations in the book; it is counter-cultural to admit that you are proud of what you are, even more difficult to ask other people to agree. But by allowing yourself to celebrate the good things about you, you begin to not only to feel good about them, but also to use them as a resource at times when you think you are not doing well.

'He is fine about being asked to do something, or not to do something, in bed.'

Men who accept being asked to do something, or to do something differently, quickly learn to drive women wild. Being able to change what you are doing in mid-stroke is a sign of real maturity! The key is to realize that being asked to change doesn't mean you are getting it wrong or that you are going to be abandoned because you are failing. Our minds have a tendency to remember failures better than successes, and to be incredibly vulnerable when they think they are getting it wrong – usually with a direct line to the penis! If your mind can see a request as a sign of trust and love in a relationship, a sign that you are actually doing well rather than failing, then it can sidestep the drooping erection, and give you sexual success instead.

Action: Next time you are asked to change what you are doing in bed, remind yourself that this gives you an opportunity to do it even better! Make a point of being enthusiastic about that, of really checking out just what is wanted and how you can supply it. Then reward yourself by allowing yourself a sexual treat. Don't turn it into a bargain – 'I'll do that if you do this' – but give yourself something special: a stunning fantasy during love-making, buying a vibrator, a sensuous bath and relaxation session. Make special pleasure your reward for learning to feel confident about giving.

'He feels he can ask for what he wants.'

The other side of the coin is to be sufficiently self-confident to ask for things without embarrassment; failure to do this leads to all kinds of horrible side-effects in bed, including loss of erection because you are not getting the stimulation you need. The myth is that if you ask for what you want you are being selfish in some way; the result is that people often feel guilty about making requests in bed and end up either complaining about doing so, or waiting until they are desperate and then demanding something angrily. Neither of these options are nearly as sexually effective as a direct request.

Action: Next time you know you want something different in bed, ask for it. Check first that you are really relaxed; if not, your body language or your voice may send out anxious signals. Remind yourself that you have a right to ask and that, if you are refused, this is not a put-down. Have at the back of your mind another alternative in the event your suggestion isn't acceptable. As you ask for what you want, really get in touch with how sexually excited you would be if your request were granted, how much that would turn you on. Who could resist, if they really understood how aroused you would get if they gave you what you wanted? To take things further, join an assertiveness course – though its reputation is for helping women, classes are often mixed or men-only, and help you to ask clearly and without 'running a number' for what you really want.

'He is at ease with closeness and intimacy.'

Most of us feel uneasy if other people come too close to us physically or emotionally. There is a particular zone in the body, called the intimacy zone; it could be your stomach, back, shoulders, thighs. This zone gets tense if someone moves too close or starts being too emotional – yet we often override the comfort zone during sex, when sheer pleasure drives us into each other's arms. Then, we suddenly realize that we are being too intimate and panic, pushing people away emotionally or even literally. This can happen even in the longest-term relationships; one interviewee told us of feeling panic, 'as if I were going to be suffocated', if his wife started to cry. In its worst manifestation, being ill at ease with intimacy can kill desire, erection and the ability to come.

Action: If you are wary of intimacy, take it slowly; expect to feel a bit uneasy when faced with emotional closeness. First, identify which part of your body is the intimacy zone where you feel this unease – stomach, back, shoulders? Then start to be aware, in bed, if this intimacy zone is being invaded. Whenever you feel an intrusion – someone moving too close for comfort, someone bursting into tears near you – try the full body relaxation that we outline in Chapter 15, along with keeping eye contact. Allow yourself to be more and more relaxed when this happens and, over several occasions, gradually respond to an intrusion by being welcoming and open, by offering a hug or a willingness to listen. The twist is this: long term, your action will not invite more intrusion. In fact, the exact opposite: ultimately, if welcomed, the other person is more likely to relax and so be more able in the long run to give you the space that you need.

BUILDING A SUPERVIRILE PERSONALITY

'Lots of emotion, showing whatever he feels...'

Emotion enhances sex and makes it meaningful. In addition, withholding your emotions leads to an actual anaesthetization of your physical feelings. So admitting to what you are feeling in bed will not only create an atmosphere of relaxation and security, but will allow you to experience more sensation. Your first challenge then is to raise the pleasure level by saying that you are getting turned on, moan your pleasure or murmur words of love. Admitting that you are tearful, which people often are near orgasm, may take a bit more practice. The real crunch, separating the men from the boys, is for men to admit that they are scared, particularly if they have failed to get an erection last time. Remember that most women will react much better to your true feelings than to any kind of machismo. It is not the technical failure that turns women off, but the attempt to hide your feelings.

Action: Next time you are in bed, try making a little more noise. No words yet, just relax your facial muscles and let the noise come out. After a few occasions, put words to the noise: 'wonderful, again, scary'. Next time, include the word 'I' in what you say: 'I love that, I love you, I think I'm going to come, I'm worried I'm not going to come'. Let your emotion show through, more and more.

'He lets go when he's aroused, doesn't hang on to control all the time.'

Too many men think that they need to be in charge all the time, either of their own pleasure or of the sex act. This can even turn into 'spectatoring', a constant inner dialogue, an awareness of watching oneself from the outside rather than getting in there and enjoying. This is death not only to sexual enjoyment but also to anything that involves performance as, when you act the role of spectator, you will naturally tend to criticize yourself. Having the self-confidence really to experience sensations from the inside during times when you are aroused will not only be more pleasurable for you, but will also create a more relaxed atmosphere in bed. But it is difficult sometimes; one client described 'letting go' as quite unsafe, 'like going down a slide'. You don't know what might happen, as your mind allows your body to take over.

Action: Try experimenting with different kinds of letting go. First, go on a slide, go on a trampoline, go to a funfair and go on the rides. When in bed, practise accepting as much pleasure as you can, focusing your attention on each sense in turn and imagining the sensation increasing and increasing. Allow yourself to be passive in bed; arrange with your partner that, this time, you will offer nothing back but will allow her to pleasure you completely. Then lie back and enjoy it – although if scared feelings do arise, express them, and share them with your partner.

'He's not fazed if it doesn't work occasionally.'

If you ever suffer from not being able to get it up, this is the key problem, the underpinning of all impotence issues – the panic of performance anxiety. First, if something goes wrong (no desire, no erection, no orgasm for you, or your partner...) you feel bad at the time. Then, when you think about next time, you imagine it happening again and feel worse. What if the problems continue; my partner might not want me any more? After a while, the anxiety about the failure is greater than the anxiety about not bothering, and what was a case of not being able to get it up becomes a case of loss of desire.

Action: If something does go wrong, go back to simply playing. Puncture the tension by laughing about it. If you start panicking about next time, again relax. Try putting a ban on intercourse for a whole week and just cuddling. In the long term, train yourself to play rather than perform; spend time with the kids, take time off, start noticing that there are other things in life but performance. A second, more challenging idea is this: take time on your own one day to compose two mental messages. The first should be from yourself to your penis, expressing all the things that you think and feel about it, particularly at times when it doesn't do what you want it to. If your message is like the ones most men construct when asked to do this exercise, it will provide you with a great deal of insight about how you subconsciously berate your poor maligned organ! Next, send a message back, from your penis to yourself, maybe defending itself, maybe pointing out ways in which you may block it from doing what it wants to do. This exploration will mean you never see your penis, or your performance, in the same light ever again!

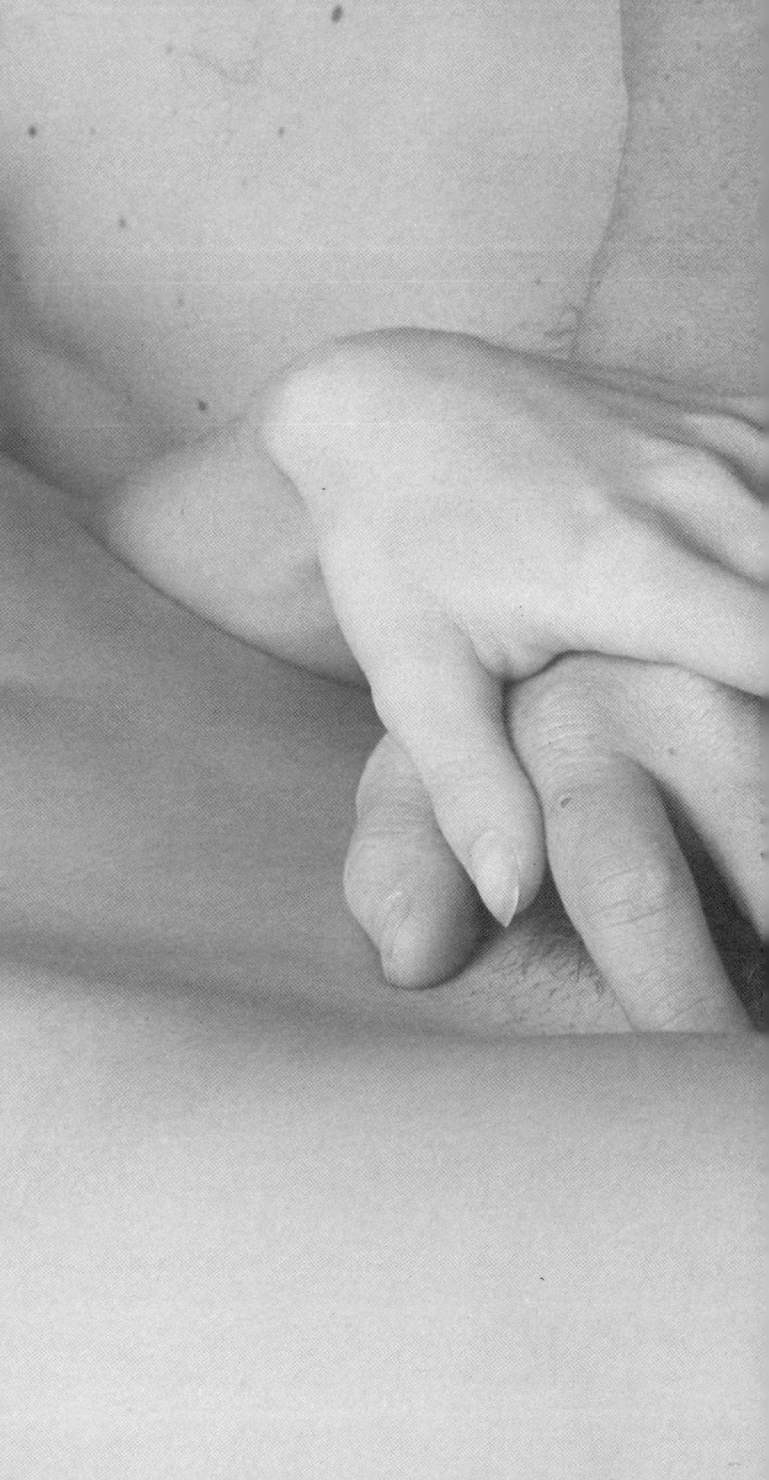

Building a Supervirile Personality

'No hang-ups, does anything, shares fantasies, tries different things.'

Open-mindedness is the key to long-lasting and interesting sexuality. First, being able to accept sex without any guilt or hang-ups, sweat, blood, tears and all, makes love-making a rewarding experience in itself, as you enter wholeheartedly into the experience without any physical pulling back. Secondly, being able to go on from that acceptance to open-minded innovation is the way to make excitement last for ever. For it is very tempting to find out what suits you, and then stick to that, gradually narrowing down the field until in the end you have a rigid and boring ritual. Instead, have the mental energy to think up new things and then action them, as well as being at ease with the whole range of possible sexual options.

Action: Build your own self-confidence to suggest new things by doing so outside the bedroom; go to a new restaurant, experiment with cooking something new, try a different sport. Learn from these that other people may react warily but, in the end, they are often grateful that you made the first move. When you come to the bedroom, admit your embarrassment and confide your fear of freak-outs. Get relaxed with everything sex involves – explore each other's bodies fully; look, touch, smell and taste. Then find out about other sexual options to add to your repertoire, by reading books like this one, or by buying and trying some erotica or sex toys. Set sexual goals – whether that is being able to swing from the chandeliers or simply aiming to make love with the light on – and then take action!

'He's really over the moon when things go well.'

Some men sabotage themselves in bed because they can't handle success. Experts reckon that this is one of the underlying bases both of premature ejaculation (coming too soon because they are afraid of lasting longer) and delayed ejaculation (not coming at all because they are afraid of the success of orgasm). Certainly the ability to pat oneself on the back is not a key feature of the male psyche! But really enjoying success in bed means that can be built upon next time.

Action: Check out other places in your life where you are wary of celebrating success. Start setting yourself a programme of celebration, indulging in birthday presents, end-of-the-project parties, and pay-rise extravaganzas. Then watch the celebration factor gradually insinuate itself into your love-making. Pop champagne in the fridge for afterwards. Give each other presents after a particularly good session. Bounce on the bed to celebrate the best orgasm ever in the history of the world.

Try each of the above explorations for a few weeks; then allow it to integrate, and move on after a month or so to another exploration you are attracted to. In the end, you will notice the results affecting the whole way you see yourself, your sex life and your relationships.

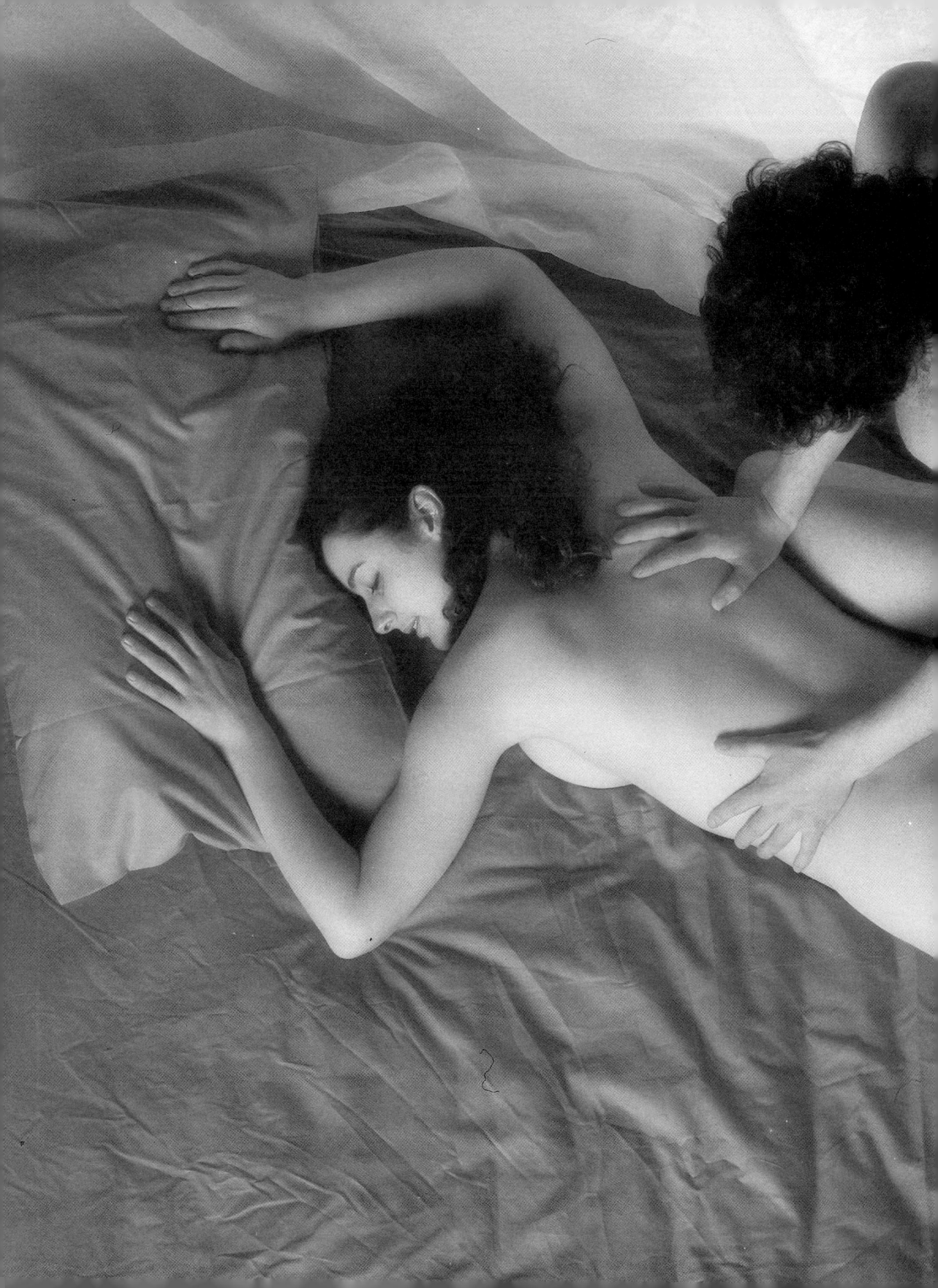

Part III

Relationship Supervirility

Understanding Your Partner

Sexuality is about relationships. Our individual bodies and minds give us pleasure, and we can certainly masturbate alone with a great deal of enjoyment. But for real fulfilment and potential, we turn to our partner.

In addition, the success of our love-making is inextricably linked with our relationship because, in sex, each one of us is deeply affected by the other. If one of us draws back, the other will be wary; if one of us feels loving, the other will respond. If one of us climaxes joyously, then that will make the other happy, too.

So, if we are really committed to enhancing our sexuality, we must also be committed to exploring our relationship; we need to examine our interactions with our partner in order to really make sure that they are supporting our Supervirility.

A good first step is understanding your partner. For although in the past three decades, since the advent of the Pill, sexual choice and women's lib, men and women have moved far closer together than ever before in their attitudes to sex; nevertheless the genders are still very different. On top of this, though you and your partner may well have grown increasingly close over the years, you are still very different people. And, finally, though love grows, time spent together may actually have forced you to develop independently. However much you think you know what your partner thinks and feels, constant updating is essential if you are to create love-making that really works.

Your Partner's Past

Like you, your partner will have gained her basic personality from the experiences and events in her past, particularly early childhood. She will have received both direct and indirect messages about sex not only from her own explorations into how her body works, but also from people around her – parents, religious leaders, friends, peers, sexual partners. Like you, she will probably have ended up with a mixture of good and bad feelings about sex. Together, within your relationship, you will probably have already reassured each other, opened doorways to non-guilty pleasure, and helped each other build sexual skill. You will probably already be able to identify with your partner, sexually and emotionally, on a deep level.

But what about where your experiences differ? What about when your approach and that of your partner don't match? Remember as you read this chapter that we are offering only generalizations; some of these comments may not be true about your partner, or only true some of the time.

- Even from her early childhood, your partner will probably have been told that, in order to be OK, she must look physically pleasing. The positive side of this is that she, far more than you, will constantly strive to keep looking good. But, as she gets older and child-bearing thickens her waist, or the menopause brings on wrinkles and grey hair, she may start losing confidence, and start to believe that she isn't a sexual person any longer. She may need reassurance that she is still attractive, if she is to maintain her desire.

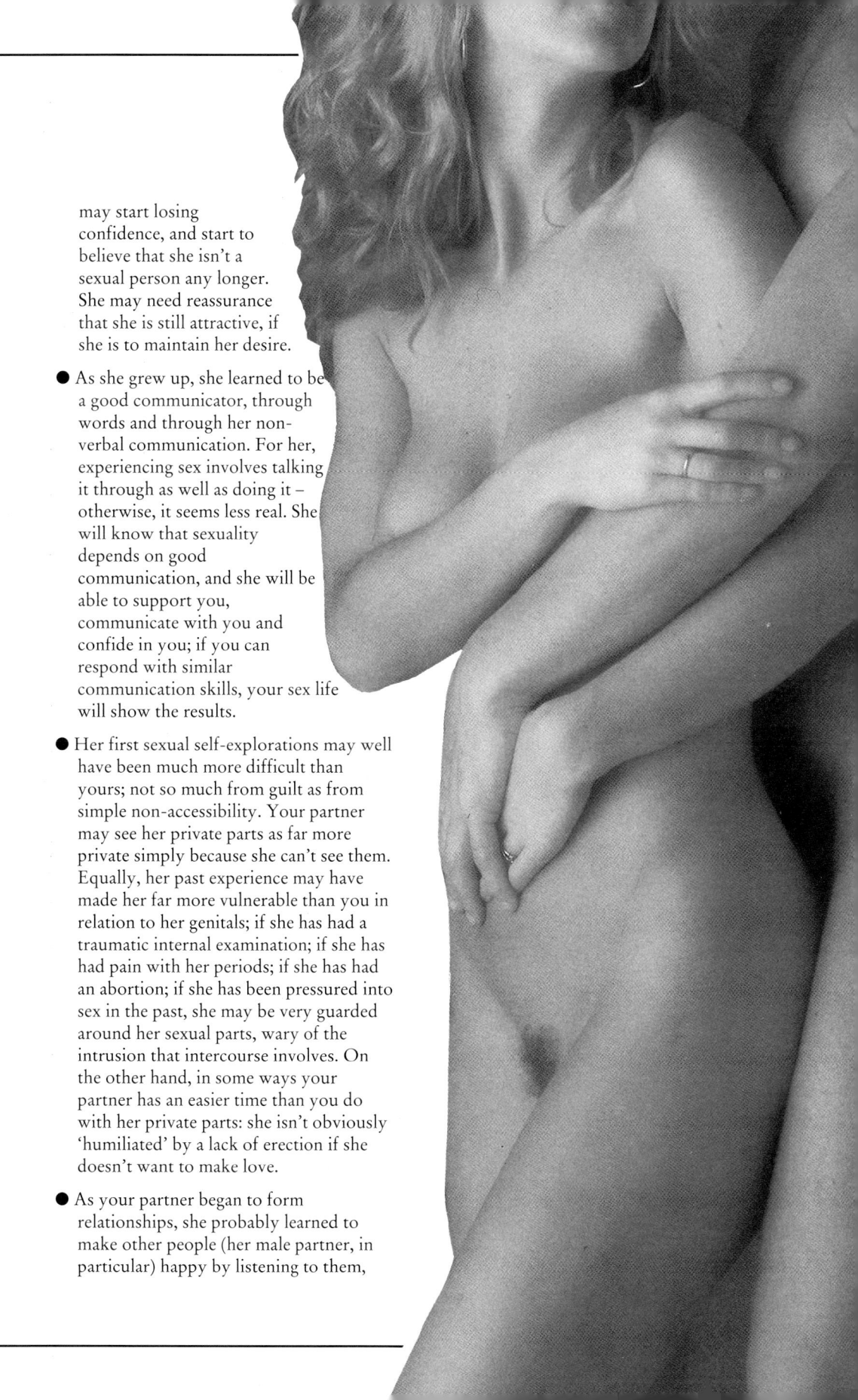

- As she grew up, she learned to be a good communicator, through words and through her non-verbal communication. For her, experiencing sex involves talking it through as well as doing it – otherwise, it seems less real. She will know that sexuality depends on good communication, and she will be able to support you, communicate with you and confide in you; if you can respond with similar communication skills, your sex life will show the results.

- Her first sexual self-explorations may well have been much more difficult than yours; not so much from guilt as from simple non-accessibility. Your partner may see her private parts as far more private simply because she can't see them. Equally, her past experience may have made her far more vulnerable than you in relation to her genitals; if she has had a traumatic internal examination; if she has had pain with her periods; if she has had an abortion; if she has been pressured into sex in the past, she may be very guarded around her sexual parts, wary of the intrusion that intercourse involves. On the other hand, in some ways your partner has an easier time than you do with her private parts: she isn't obviously 'humiliated' by a lack of erection if she doesn't want to make love.

- As your partner began to form relationships, she probably learned to make other people (her male partner, in particular) happy by listening to them, checking out what they want and then supplying that. Whereas you have been taught to perform, she has probably been taught to please. Whereas you have been taught to be active, she may have been taught to be passive. So she may be totally at ease giving you time and attention, able to support you even when (perhaps particularly when) things go wrong in bed. She is far less likely than you to be worried about performance, and she may well be happy to go with what you want sexually, even if she does not particularly get pleasure from it. On the other hand, she may find it difficult to know what she wants, or to express her dissatisfaction; she may feel unable to initiate sex or to make requests in bed. She may feel unable to take action if she is unhappy with what is happening and, if so, she may, without knowing it, also be feeling powerless and angry. As a result, she may on occasions want to undermine you, or hurt you emotionally – showing this in irritation, put-downs, rows and perhaps even loss of desire.

- Your partner will have had more opportunity than you have had to develop emotions; whereas you will have been encouraged to *act*, she will tend to *feel*, particularly in bed, where sex and emotions are for her often indivisible. This means that her emotions need exercise, and just as some men feel uneasy if they don't regularly use their bodies in sport or physical exertion, she may feel uncomfortable if she doesn't express her emotion. She may also be more emotionally vulnerable, and will certainly feel hurt if you are unable to respond to her expression of feelings – conversely, she is far more able to give sex the emotional dimension that makes it whole.

LIFE CHANGES

You can probably already begin to see how your partner's approach to life can crucially affect your success in bed together. You may already be linking certain sexual blocks between you with the differences in approach you each have. There is, however, a further element that you need to bear in mind when analysing your relationship. Your partner's attitude to sex will be affected by key life changes, particularly those which relate to her sexuality. The woman you first met may not, in fact, be the woman you are now committed to, because she herself will have undergone these changes. So the woman you now have sex with may need different understanding, different support and different expressions of love from the woman you first went to bed with.

Some of the crucial life changes are listed below.

- **Losing her virginity.** Still generally regarded as a key experience for a woman, this is more likely to be significant for your partner than the equivalent experience was for you. If it was unwilling or painful, she may even now find it difficult to relax during sex, and have an in-built anxiety which can be triggered – in much the same way as the failure of your erection can – if something unpleasant happens in sex. If losing her virginity was loving and wonderful, your partner will have built on that foundation to create a positive sex life.

- **Traumatic sexual experiences.** Incest or rape can affect a woman in the same way as they would a man. They can also lead to her blaming herself for what has happened, thus adding guilt to the uncertainty she feels around sex. Sexual operations, such as abortion, hysterectomy or treatment for cervical cancer, can also set up similar unhappy memories. For all these traumatic events, your partner may need support from you or from an outside counsellor, to become more relaxed during sex.

- **Having a baby.** There is a well-documented pattern of women losing interest in sex after child-bearing; experts disagree about whether this could be the altered hormone balance; whether life is so disrupted by a baby that there is no time or energy for sex; or whether now that sex has had its desired result, women's bodies simply put it on the back burner. On the other hand, having a baby often confirms a woman's belief in herself as a sexual person, and so increases her sexual enjoyment.

- **Not having a baby.** Equally, if a woman who really wants children is unable to have them this can be very upsetting for her sex life. She may feel so bad about herself, or about you, that she stops wanting sex. She may feel so desperate and anxious that sex becomes an unhappy experience. If, in the end, children are not a possibility, then depression may strike for both of you, and seriously disrupt your love-making. On the other hand, if you decide not to have children, or adapt to not having any, the freedom to develop your relationship together can mean that your sex life is more active than that of a couple who do have a family.

- **The midlife crisis.** Menopause itself, when periods and child-bearing ability stops, can lead to some very specific sexual changes for a woman: a sharp decline in sex hormones; a reduction in lubrication, making intercourse more difficult; an increase in the signs of ageing making her feel less desirable; a decline in sex drive. On the other hand, not having to worry about contraception may mean that sex is more relaxed than it ever has been before. Also, having her existing family leave home, thus releasing her to start work or pursue her own interests, can mean that midlife is the time when a woman feels best about herself – and this confidence will spill over into love-making.

SEXUAL MISMATCHES

There is a final sexual issue which may well be influencing your relationship, here and now. This element is nothing to do with you and everything to do with your biology.

Perhaps the most revolutionary sexual discovery over the past twenty years, first brought to public notice in the controversial *Hite Report*, is that what works for a man and what works for a woman during love-making can actually be totally different. In some cases, for many couples, male and female sexual cycles don't quite match; she takes a long time to get aroused, and he meanwhile is eager to come.

As he comes and wants to stop, she is ready for her next three orgasms. Equally, the most exciting movements and actions for a man may be biologically irrelevant for his partner; penetration may not touch her sensitive spots, and so no amount of intercourse will give her the pleasure it gives him. We explore in Part IV the sexual techniques you can use to solve this dilemma within your partnership. Here, however, we look at what you may need to understand about how this issue affects your partner.

First, of course, if this mismatch of patterns is true for your partner, as it is for many women, then things that are important for you in sex are likely to be unimportant for her. Your penis size, as we have stated earlier, will be irrelevant. Your stamina in thrusting, your ability to last a long time, your performance during intercourse – all these will be of far less interest to her than your willingness to cuddle, touch and stroke, to lick and caress, to perform manual and oral sex.

Secondly, you need to look at whether these mismatches have, over the years, widened or narrowed the gap between you and your partner. The chances are that, when you met, any mismatch in your needs was neither apparent nor important, for three reasons. Sheer desire to make love may have overridden any intrinsic problems. Your partner may have liked simply being close to you and been able to ignore the fact that her sexual pleasure was not all that high. Finally, and most importantly, you probably spent a lot more time touching, licking, arousing, before intercourse – foreplay which increases the proportion of directly pleasurable activity for your partner.

Perhaps, as your relationship developed, the need for the 'real' sex of intercourse backed up; earlier and earlier, you moved to straightforward intercourse, without the preliminaries that your partner may have needed. Your partner may have been totally happy that, although for her things weren't so good physically, your physical satisfaction made it worthwhile. But, even so, time after time of not quite enjoying it or not quite coming may have built up a reservoir of disappointment and consequent anger that now affects the whole of her attitude to sex.

The alternative, which many couples do achieve, is that over the years you have discovered ways of moving, ways of penetrating, ways of touching or ways of taking orgasm that create equal pleasure for you both. In this case, or if your partner is a woman whose biology allows her to feel direct stimulation during intercourse, then over the years her pleasure will have increased – and so will her satisfaction.

We will be exploring in much greater detail in Chapter 12 the ways that your partner and you together can work around any incompatibilities. The issue here is to realize that you should understand that your partner's needs in bed may be different from yours – and realize that, if she is less arousable than she used to be, this mismatch may be the reason.

FINDING OUT

Here is an exploration for you to do together in order to update your understanding of each other and make it relevant to your love life today.

This is the first exercise in the book in which you do need to involve your partner – although, from now on, there will be more and more of these exercises. So here is a rider about your partner being involved: she may have doubts, for a number of reasons.

- **She may be afraid.** She may fear that if the explorations don't work, and your sex life doesn't improve, she will get the blame. Or, she may be scared of exploring the relationship in case you both find out things you'd rather not know. She will need to be reassured by you that the first of these will not happen, and that the second is something your partnership can cope with and survive.

- **Your partner may no longer be motivated to work on the relationship.** We have said that this is not a book you would read if you thought your relationship was on the rocks. But it could be that your partner is at the end of her commitment, and that this is what is stopping you getting your sex life back. If so, you should really be facing up to that fact.

- **Your partner may be scared that your sex life will improve.** This may seem strange, but it could be that your relationship is working better for your partner without an enhanced sex life. Perhaps because you have a problem, she gets to support and mother you, and she likes doing that. Perhaps underneath everything, she is so angry at you that she wants you to fail, particularly in bed. Perhaps at present she doesn't want to make love – and sees these explorations as just more pressure on her. Perhaps what you see as a problem (lack of erection, delayed ejaculation) is a benefit for her (she misses out on penetration but gets oral sex instead; she has much more intercourse and comes more often).

Talk through with your partner her reasons for feeling as she does. A better sex life for you has to involve a better sex life for your partner, and she may need to know that. If you can do these explorations together, regard that as your first (and only really essential) step forward; if you both really want to enhance the relationship, then you will get what you want.

Take it in turns to talk through this list of headings, missing out those that aren't relevant. Take one heading at a time, with first one of you then the other answering fully – the silent partner is able to ask questions, but not interrupt with comments or titbits of his or her own. Of course, if one or the other of you gets emotional, then take time out to comfort or to cuddle. If talking seems too challenging, write your answers down and give them to each other to read.

1. Tell me about your very first sexual memory? What happened? How did you feel? Was it a good or a negative experience – do you think it still affects you today?

2. Tell me about your childhood, what people taught you about sex, nudity, love relationships, from what they said and did? What sort of sexual relationship do you think your parents had? Did you have any sexual crises when you were little? How did you learn the facts of life – and was what you learned correct?

3. (For her) When did you first start your periods? What was it like and how did you feel? (For him) When did you first have a wet dream or an ejaculation? What was it like and how did you feel?

4. When did you first masturbate? Did it feel good? Were you ever found out, and what did that feel like?

5. How did you feel about the way you looked when you were growing up? Did you see yourself as sexually attractive?

6. What was your first sexual experience? What about your first kiss? Your first heavy petting session?

7. How did you lose your virginity? Was it a good experience? Was it pleasurable? How would you have liked it to be different? Do you think it has affected your sex life now?

8. What memories do you have of past sexual partners; what did they teach you, both good and bad lessons, about sex? (Avoid this question if there is tension between you about past relationships.)

9. Have you had any upsetting sexual experiences: unwilling sex; operations or injuries to sexual parts of you? Do you feel that they are still affecting love-making for us? (If so, then you may want to seek professional help.)

10. (For both of you) How does having children/not having children affect sex for you, and how you see yourself as a sexual person because of that?

11. (For both of you) How does the midlife crisis affect your sex life?

12. (for both of you) How do you feel about sex now? (If you want to talk about how it could be better, turn to the exploration in Chapter 14.)

Now you have begun to explore you will probably want to continue to update your knowledge regularly. Add to it, too, by reading accounts of how others feel about sex and relationships, such as the *Hite Report* for you, or the *Hite Report on Men* for her. Make sure that you are aware of how women in general, and your partner in particular, thinks and feels – not only in bed, but in the more general context of your relationship – and you will find your sex life beginning to reflect your greater understanding.

SUPERVIRILITY

WHEN YOUR LOVE BLOCKS YOUR LUST
11

On a very basic level, it is your interaction with your partner that determines how much pleasure you get from sex. We all accept that loving sex is more worthwhile – but in a literal, physiological sense, the emotions you feel about each other affect your body state and movement. If irritation is the emotion of which you are most aware, this can actually stop you from sensing as clearly; stifled anger can anaesthetize your sensations so that you don't feel as much; conversely, the relaxation that security and love bring means that you are able to experience more pleasure on a minute-to-minute level.

This chapter faces head on the current state of your relationship and how that has built up over the years. It explores what you may be thinking and feeling about each other as a couple, and how this may be affecting your Supervirility.

As you read, bear in mind that most people who do have sexual blocks linked with their relationship are not on the brink of destruction. They don't want to leave, they don't hate each other, they are committed to their relationship and their families. If they weren't, lack of desire wouldn't bother them in the least. It is the couples who still love each other – for whom a sexual block is preventing the euphoria that they know they can have – who are most conscious of sexual issues, and most willing to work on them. As Marj Thoburn, the Head of Sex Therapy at the British organization RELATE (formerly the National Marriage Guidance Council), commented to us when we spoke to her, 'You don't have to have a relationship problem to have a sexual problem.'

Nevertheless, this may be a hard chapter to work through. If you begin to recognize that your relationship needs changing in order to enhance your sexuality, you may be tempted to turn the page. If you are tempted, please remember that the better your interaction with your partner, the better your experience of sex will be.

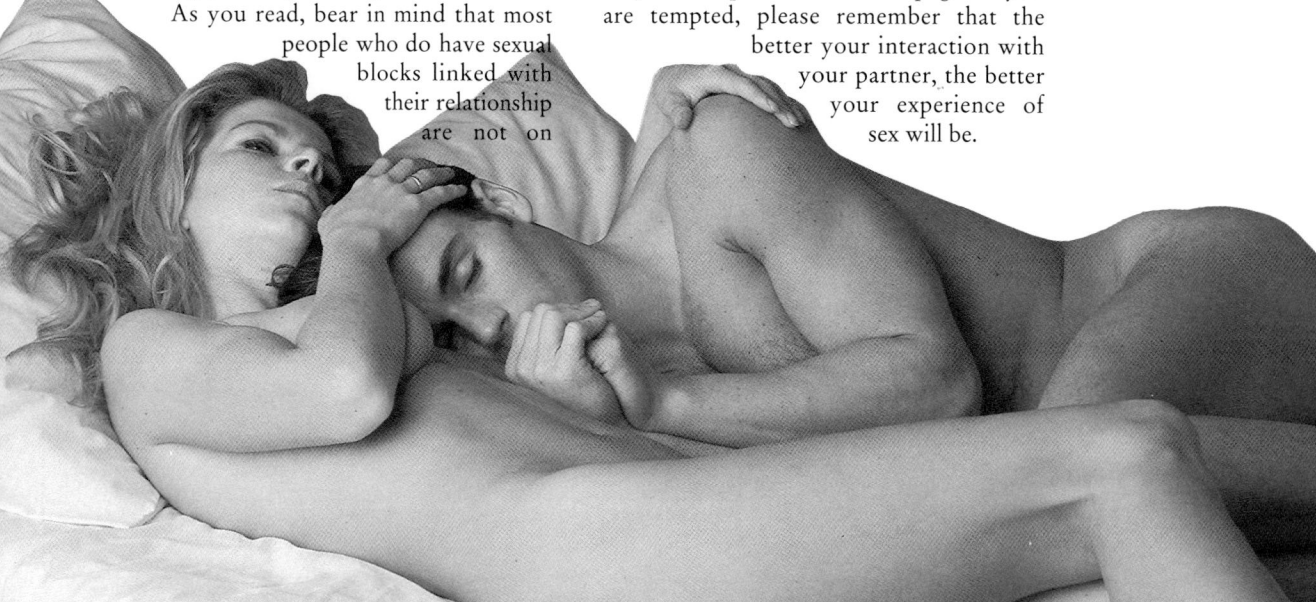

What Underlies Your Relationship?

Undoubtedly, when you met, you were in love and in lust. Whether you met your partner a few months, years or decades ago, the start was wonderful, positive and hopeful – or you would not have fallen for each other.

However you began your relationship, you will, over the time you are together, have started to set up patterns of interaction between you that both added to and subtracted from the first flush of love. The positive elements of these patterns normally allow us to develop good communication, negotiation skills, trust, security and mutual effectiveness; they lead us into affection, working together as a couple, lifelong commitment, and they make love-making a comfortable and pleasurable exercise. The negative elements create misunderstanding, lack of trust, instability, disillusionment; they create resentment, disharmony and a tendency to undermine each other, and they make love-making far less likely, perhaps boring, sometimes traumatic.

Some of the following points may sound familiar to you.

- As we have explained before, we all bring into our relationship our **past experiences** about sex and relationships. The negative ones, the emotional scars, make us think, feel and act in certain unhelpful ways – holding back from intimacy, being worried or performance-oriented in bed, being uptight about sex. As we stated in Chapters 6 and 10, both of you have to neutralize these past scars in order to make love to your full potential.

- Specifically, we often get attracted to others because they remind us of **key figures** in our past lives. So we may have chosen our partners because they are able to give us the love and affection we would have liked when young. This is a wonderful foundation for a relationship, and allows us to relax and feel secure in the context of our partnership. However, as many schools of psychology point out, such choices can also create real problems if we then expect from our partner the kind of all-embracing love that we expected from our parents – being there for us all the time, solving all our problems, caring for us constantly. For partners are our equals, ordinary human beings just like us. Confusing our partners with key figures in our lives, usually totally unconsciously, means that we can demand inappropriate things from them, and end up angry; anger is one of the key murderers of desire in relationships. Better by far to see our partner as an adult equal from whom we can expect ordinary, human vices and virtues.

- If we and our partners do succeed in acting like parents to each other, this leads to another problem – feeling **asexual** about each other. For it is very unlikely that we felt actively sexual about our parents (despite what some psychoanalysts claim, most of us don't actually feel lust for our father or mother). We know that the right way to feel in relation to our parents is asexual: affectionate, loving, depending, giving – but not aroused. So if we start to confuse our partner with our mother, then we stop seeing her as a lover. This can be exacerbated even further if we start a family; our partner actually becomes a mother, and so the temptation to regard her as a mother figure becomes even stronger. We need to be very clear that we are not each other's parents, and to know it is all right to feel sexual about each other again, in order for our desire to surface.

- As time passes and our relationship grows, even if we avoid the 'parent trap', it is in the course of human nature that we will not get everything we expected from our partner. It is no coincidence that the marriage service slips in the prophetic phrase 'for better or worse'; all too often, our minds seize on the 'worse' and get disillusioned. In day-to-day terms, what experts call the '**unconscious rage**' that this produces can underpin a lot of what we do, creating a tendency to blame or hit out at each other, undermine each other or withdraw from each other. It is not surprising that when taken into bed this will translate itself into a lack of desire or a withholding during love-making. In some women, it resolves itself into an emotion so strong that some psychologists have dubbed it a 'castration' wish; your partner may unconsciously want you to have problems and to fail in bed. However, if we can contact this rage and acknowledge it, turn it on its head and start focusing on the good things we get from our relationship, then love and 're-illusionment' will bring the lust back.

- There is, in all of us, usually triggered by childhood experiences, a **deep-seated terror** of being left, deserted, abandoned, unloved. However much we gloss over it, however self-sufficient we think we are, if we fall in love we do not want our partner to reject and walk out on us. So if our partnership is vital to us, we can end up secretly terrified that it will end; this terror can show itself in the relationship through anxiety, jealousy, trying to please, shutting down on feelings, not asking for what we want – or withdrawing totally so that we don't get hurt. In bed, desire is the first element to go if we are anxious, and our erection may well be the second! If we feel secure in our relationship and in our partner's love, then even sexual problems can be overcome, because we are not paralysed with terror.

- In a curious and frustrating double-bind, we can often suffer a **constant negative swing** from 'rage' to 'terror' and back again – though, of course, we are rarely aware of these feelings quite so strongly. We may begin by feeling irritated with our partner for something and so not wanting to make love; as soon as we realize we are irritated and realize, too, that this irritation is threatening our relationship, we switch to anxiety that perhaps we are failing our partner. This in turn dampens our desire. After a while, realizing that we are anxious about the relationship, we begin to get annoyed about that, and swing back again into irritation. Experts suggest that this constant negative swing can, in an established relationship, keep sex constantly at bay. If we can move out of the constant swing, then we can regain the desire we feel.

- An added element is your **response to crisis** – redundancy, a bereavement, menopause, a midlife loss of confidence, an affair. When such a crisis strikes, initially we may offer each other support. But when the dust has settled, often the impact is negative. If we are feeling vulnerable, crisis immediately ups the ante and exaggerates negative reactions. A midlife crisis which makes you insecure, may push your partner away, in bed and out of it. Her menopause, leaving her less likely to want to make love for a while, may make you feel rejected. If she goes out to work, and you feel threatened by her sudden independence, then you may become possessive and demanding and she may react by withdrawing sexually. The initial event may pass, but the impact of this sudden burst of negative feeling remains with us, and each time we get into bed together, we remember it and withdraw. If the crisis brings us closer together, however, and lets us contact the sympathy and empathy we feel for each other, then it can actually fuel our desire to make love together.

- The final twist to the whole issue of relationship affecting sexuality is that if you do get a **sexual problem**, this in itself can affect your relationship. If one of you develops a block, often in order to defend yourself against the other, then that often makes things worse. If you cannot get it up, your partner may feel angry and rejected. If she doesn't want to make love, you may both feel scared that the relationship will end. In fact, women are often far less threatened by lack of performance on the part of men than men are, so by their very understanding may defuse the situation; but sometimes they put on pressure to have sex because they need that as a statement that you still love them. If we can learn to back off when sexual problems arise, and give each other space, very often this move alone can help resolve the situation.

WHERE ARE YOU NOW?

While reading this list of relationship elements that can directly affect your sex life, you may well have been beginning to pinpoint the ones that might be affecting you. To help you focus more clearly, we offer this list of blocks, and track back their possible relationship causes. Bear in mind that no one block will have a simple explanation – and also that it may well be tied up with physical causes, your own particular mental approach, and your sexual knowledge an technique, as well as the dynamic in your relationship.

1. **Feeling lust was never there.** If desire has never really been there between you, then this is more likely due to deep-seated past issues than your particular relationship. Perhaps because of your past history, you are unable to feel true lust for someone of your partner's type – or able to feel lust at all in an intimate relationship. Some men, for example, can only feel desire for someone they do not love, such as a prostitute or a one-night stand. If this is so for you, firstly, celebrate that despite your lack of sex, your relationship is still surviving – your bond is obviously strong. You may want to turn to one-to-one counselling to clear up the buried memories and allow you to contact the lust.

2. **Shutting down desire.** Perhaps your desire has faded slowly, over the years; if so, you are not alone, as this is the most common pattern in all relationships. You will need to consider many if not all of

the elements we mention above as the root causes. You or your partner's disillusionment may be causing you to hold back your desire, or even subconsciously undermine each other's attempts at sexuality. Your dependence may be hitting you with anxiety every time you attempt to make love; you may have lost lust because you are confusing your partner with a parent. Perhaps over the years, because of unacknowledged negative emotion, you simply have stopped feeling, because emotions have become too painful – and, of course, this means stopping feeling physical sensation, too. If any of these seem true to you, you need to work to iron out feelings over the whole of your relationship.

It is very common, also, for desire to die after a particularly traumatic event: did your lack of lust start immediately after an affair or a row? If so, you need to look at just what happened then, and how you can retrace your steps.

3. **Getting bored with sex.** Perhaps you have begun your partnership with certain sexual patterns that turn you both on. But over the years, mutual inhibition has set in. Perhaps within your relationship, asking and giving have become difficult, so your repertoire becomes more and more limited. You have to learn to give, to take, to ask and to be at ease with asking. Perhaps because of hidden 'rage' you are unwilling to initiate sex, learn what the other really wants, give when it is asked for.

Alternatively, if you have unrealistic expectations of each other, or have become disillusioned, then you may feel that ordinary, loving sex is boring. You need to close the gap between what you think you want and what you actually have, to see your partner and your sex life in realistic terms and to accept them.

Finally, boredom can set in if, as we have mentioned before, your strong negative feelings for each other mean that you shut down not only on emotions but also on physical sensation. In order to begin to feel sexual sensation again, you need to learn to feel emotions, in a way that is safe and unthreatening to you.

4. **Going into a failure spiral.** If getting it up has been an issue throughout your relationship, then there is probably an underlying fear that you are not good enough for your partner. Has the relationship been based on the belief you both have that she is doing you a favour by being your partner? Are either of you convinced that you constantly need to prove something to each other?

If your impotence happened suddenly, track it back to a particular event. As we have said before, this event could be any of a number of life changes. Did you or your partner have an affair? Do you feel you let her down in some big way, or did she do something that makes you feel you have to win her back?

Equally, a simple physical cause or a one-off failure can be totally exacerbated by how you and your partner react to it. Erectile dysfunction, more than any other sexual block, can be kept going by you both pushing each other into mutual patterns of feeling bad. If you and your partner have a relationship in which you both affect each other very deeply – a pattern which, when things are going well, creates boundless potential for making each other happy – this can, when things go badly, make them even worse.

5. **Rushing towards climax.** If you have always come too soon, then this is likely to be the result of past experiences, before you met your partner. If you are experiencing a sudden burst of coming too soon, then look closely at whether some event has made you angry with your partner or with yourself, leading you to undermine your success or to want to take revenge on her by cutting short her pleasure.

   In general, too, look at what you regard as coming too soon; does your partner agree, or is she happy with the pace you set? Alternatively, have you only just realized that the length of time you originally saw as suitable in intercourse is not satisfactory for her; if so, you may be feeling under pressure to last longer and, in totally understandable rebellion, are coming to your timetable rather than anyone else's. If you feel that your premature ejaculation is due to relationship issues, particularly if you can link them back to a particular event, you need to clear the anger that may be building up between you.

6. **Holding back from climax.** Feeling unable to come easily is often due to early traumatic events. But relationships too can add to this feeling. Perhaps you are not secure enough in your partnership to let go – or perhaps you feel overwhelmed by your partner and so want to stay in control of your own sexuality. In particular, if your partner tends to nag or to put strong limits round you, you may feel that choosing to come when you want is a way to demonstrate that you are still in charge of your body, if not of your relationship.

   Equally, your partnership can add to your feeling of not deserving pleasure or success. If you get into a dynamic with your partner of feeling criticized or not quite good enough, this may once again lead you to deny yourself pleasure by not coming. In all these situations, you need to look in general terms at how your relationship is building or undermining your self-esteem.

7. **When she feels bad too.** Although this is a book about ironing out your sexual issues, it must be obvious that, if your partner has a sexual block, that will affect you as well. Of course, it is possible for you alone to take pleasure but, in the long term, your partner's dissatisfaction with this will insinuate itself into your sex life, at the very least diminishing the wish to make love. It is worthwhile talking through with your partner what blocks she may be feeling – an inability to orgasm, a wariness about penetration, or diminished desire.

   Of course, all these blocks may be due to events that happened well before you met and, if so, as we suggested in Chapter 10, talking these through with you or going to one-to-one counselling will help. But, just as your sexual blocks may be reflecting mismatches within the relationship, so may your partner's. She may be angry, and be blocking you out of her life by blocking you from her vagina; she may be fearful of being left, and so be wary of letting go sufficiently to feel pleasure. Bearing in mind that your enjoyment is dependent on hers, and vice versa, you need to encourage her to work on ironing out any negativity in your relationship.

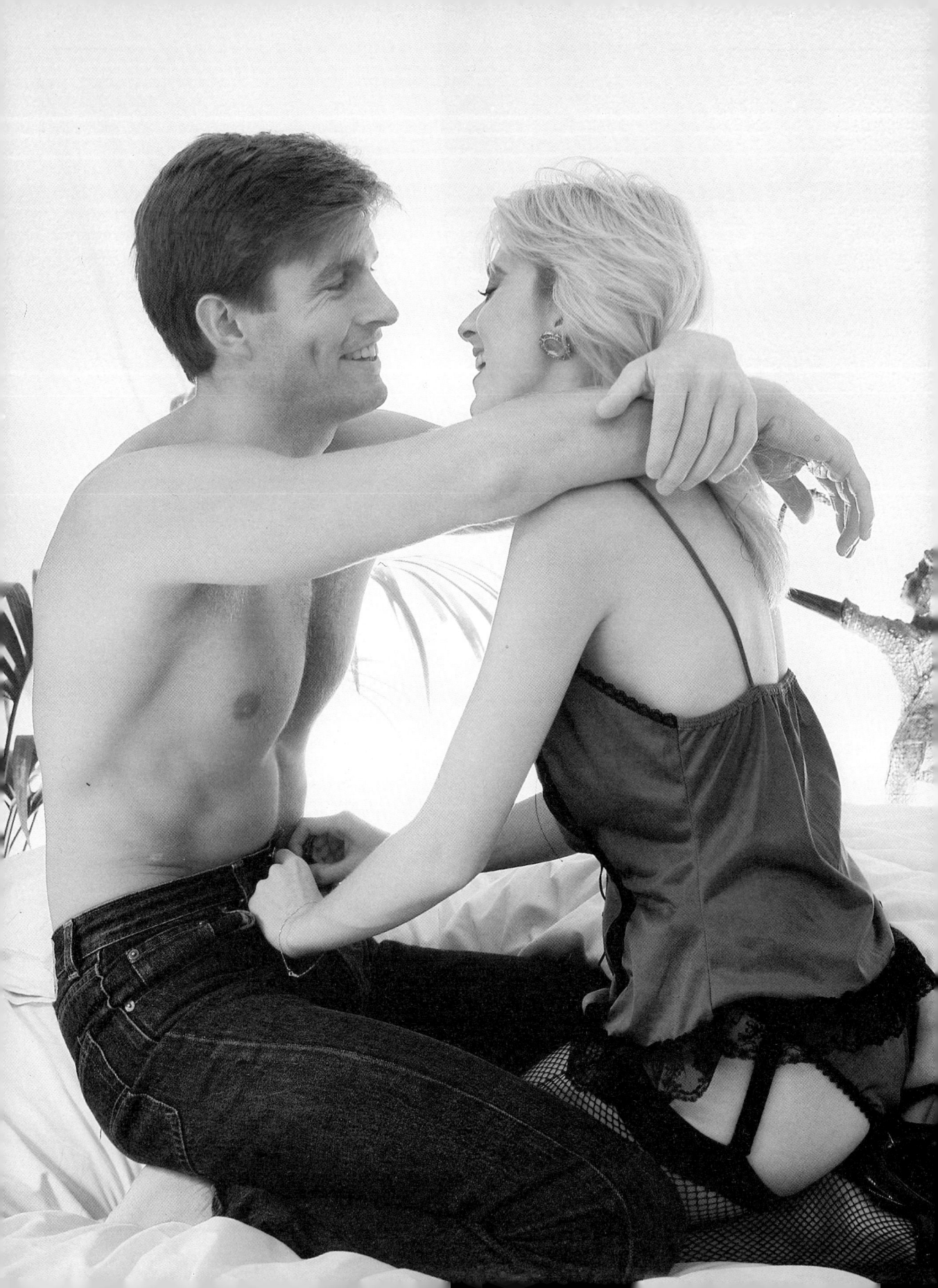

Bridging the Gap

This chapter has outlined some dynamics in your relationship that may be blocking your sexual fulfilment. In the following chapter, we offer practical suggestions to resolve these issues. This action plan acts as a bridge between analysing the blocks and dissolving them. It guides you towards identifying exactly which issues from this chapter you should be working on next – although, in fact, most relationships will benefit from working on all eight issues.

Read the following questions. Your partner should do the same, separately; when you have finished, there is no need to tell each other the answers, although you can do if you think it useful. But you will need to confide in each other which parts of the next chapter you think you should be attending to.

1. Clearing the past.
Do you feel that key events in the past still hang over your head?

Do you and your partner find it hard to forgive and forget?

2. Avoiding overdependency.
Do you find yourself thinking of your partner as a parent or sibling figure rather than as a lover?

Do you ever feel uncomfortable making love because it feels wrong to be so intimate with your partner?

3. Reducing rage.
Do you sometimes feel illogical rage against your partner for not fulfilling your needs?

Do you ever feel you want to hurt your partner emotionally, even though you love her?

4. Developing trust.
Do you ever panic in case your partner might leave, however illogical that thought might be?

Do you often feel that you are not good enough for your partner?

5. Contacting the feelings.
Do you find that you are consistently less emotional about your relationship as time passes?

Do you find yourself not mentioning things you feel strongly about because you are scared of the consequences?

6. Talking it through.
Do you find yourself talking less and less about your thoughts and feelings as time goes on?

Do you feel nervous about asking for what you want in the relationship?

7. Problem-solving.
Do crises and problems make you feel drained and hopeless?

Do you find yourself constantly at loggerheads about decisions?

8. Setting goals.
Do you tend to make plans separately rather than talking them through together?

Do you find it difficult to contact the thought of a bright future together?

If you answered yes to any of these questions, then that indicates an area of vulnerability; when you turn to Chapter 12, then you should be working on the issue your 'yes' answer pinpoints.

Finally, be reassured that all the issues we mention in this chapter are normal; what *is* abnormal is finding a couple who do not suffer any of them. All these patterns are a sign of being human!

SUPERVIRILITY

BUILDING A SUPERVIRILE RELATIONSHIP

12

You will already have established by reading Chapter 11 the areas in your relationship that you want to enhance. Each of the sections below explains the goal to set yourselves and some practical exercises for achieving them. Choose just one area to begin with, and take a few weeks to explore it. Then move on to the next area. As with all suggestions in this book, if you feel an exploration isn't right for you, stop at once and move on to the next one.

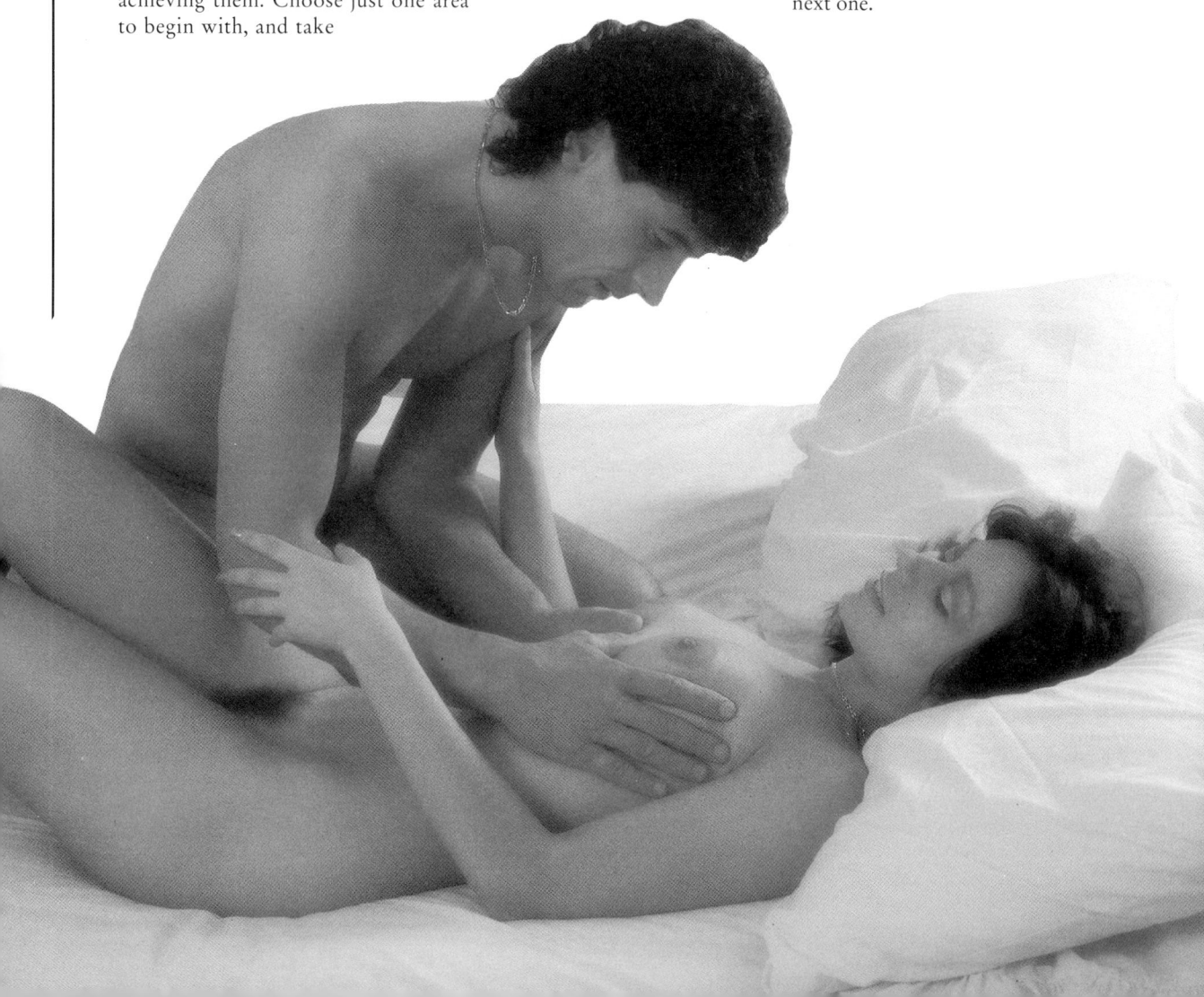

CLEARING THE PAST FOR A SEXUAL FUTURE

As we have said before, both you and your partner should aim to clear away any past distress to be at your best in this present relationship. Such distress may be holding back your desire as well as creating specific sexual blocks. You have had a chance to do this for your own personal past in Part II; your partner may also want to complete those explorations for herself. And it may be, in the case of rape or other sexual trauma, that she needs your support to go and find professional help to clear up that horror for her.

There may be some things, however, that lie between you, that you need to sort out yourselves: a past affair that is never talked about, a previous abortion that you both still regret.

Try this exploration. Sit opposite each other, perhaps on the bed, perhaps holding hands. Let the first person begin with the words 'What I really want to say to you about (the issue between you) is.' The other person should listen without interrupting until the first person has finished speaking. The listener should then repeat back what he or she understands the speaker to have said; if the listener gets it wrong, the speaker needs to correct them. Only when the listener really seems to have understood the speaker can he or she go on to make their own comment or respond to what has been said or make a new point of their own.

This exploration is a real blockbuster; it can allow you to be totally truthful with each other, to really understand how the other person feels, to start to sympathize with each other again over that issue. It can also be very difficult not to get angry, or want to interrupt. Stick with just listening; it will be worth it. If you have to stop because you are too upset, take time to calm down and then continue. Keep going, maybe even on more than one occasion, until you really feel you have understood each other. Then, you will be able to forgive.

AVOIDING OVERDEPENDENCY

As we explained in Chapter 11, expecting each other to act as parent figures can lead to fading desire, not only through resentment when you fail to meet all each other's needs, but also through confusion as you begin to feel only child–parent affection for each other. If you feel that you are losing desire the more close to and dependent you get on your partner, then you should begin by acknowledging that this is what is happening. Your goal should be to make clear that your partner is your lover, not your parent, friend or teacher. These are important roles within a relationship – but the sexual element in your partnership also needs to be strong.

Do this exploration separately from your partner. Begin by choosing three key figures in your early life – people on whom you depended, though you may have felt resentful of them, too. Write down all the ways that your partner is similar to these people, in looks, personality, attitudes, background. Be specific – if your partner and your father both had hazel eyes, then say so. If your partner and your mother both looked after you when you were ill, put that down.

Then list all the main differences you recognize about your partner and these three people: different genders, age, looks, character, approach. Again, be as specific as you can be. Aim to become clearer and clearer about how your partner and these people are not the same.

Think through what you have discovered; tell your partner about it, becoming even more aware of the distinctions between her and the key figures in your early life. As you build your own self-esteem (see Chapter 9) and become more secure in yourself, you will find yourself more able to react to your partner in appropriate ways. This exploration is just the first step in clearing the confusion.

Reducing sexual rage by clarifying expectations

The 'rage' that psychologists describe comes from disillusionment when our partner fails to do what we expect them to, or does something we don't want; it can underpin all kinds of sexual blocks on both your sides by creating withdrawal and anxiety.

Most often such disillusionment happens when we are unclear with each other about our 'contract', what we really expect from each other. We may totally agree about joint bank accounts, but still assume that our partner knows that extravagance is a hanging offence – while they think being relaxed about money is vital in a good relationship. Your goal here should be to be crystal clear with each other from now on about what you expect on every level. Particularly, be clear when you are expecting your partner to be utterly perfect, as a perfect parent would be – because this expectation is doomed to failure and must be changed.

Spend time together checking out your relationship expectations under the following headings. Don't argue about whether each of you is right to expect these things; what is important is to communicate, understand and begin to realize where the miscommunications lie.

- First check out general expectations – 'What I feel it is vital for you/me to do/not do about the house, about work, around money, about each other's parents, about the children, about friends, about being truthful, about conflict, about emotions, about time together.'

- Then check out ways in which you may be expecting your partner to be a perfect parent to you. 'I expected my mother and father to and, in the same way, I expect you to.'

- In particular, check out your sexual expectations: 'What I feel it is vital for you/me to do/not do about initiating sex, about the right time and place, about asking and getting, about how long it can last, about who has the orgasms, about whether erection or penetration are important, about oral sex and manual masturbation, about responsibility for orgasms, about making suggestions and innovations.'

It may take a great deal of talking through to bring all your expectations out into the open, but you will discover many miscommunications; after that, even if you need to discuss and negotiate on what happens, you are at least working from commonly understood ground.

Developing sexual trust that you will be neither hurt nor abandoned

If we have had bad times, then we may be mistrustful in our relationship; if we have had good times, we may still be insecure, fearing that our partner may leave because we do not believe anyone could really care for us long term. Particularly, if our parents have not been there for us as much as we wanted during childhood, we may panic, albeit unconsciously. This can result in anxiety-triggered loss of desire for both of you; for you as a man it may also lead to erectile difficulty or delayed ejaculation. Your goal should be to learn to trust in each other even more.

First, spend some time doing activities that depend on you supporting each other. Examples could be rowing on a lake, going skating together or playing together on a trampoline. These may seem like play, but if you concentrate on physically supporting each other, and on taking the emphasis off sheer performance, you will soon learn to rely on the other one to be there for you.

Secondly, practise really understanding each other on a deep level. When you are safe together, perhaps in bed, choose an incident that was key for one or the other of you and that involves a lot of physical emotion and sensation. Our favourite example of this was a woman describing to her husband the pain and ecstasy involved in giving birth to their baby. Take the time to describe the incident so vividly that the other one can really imagine not only being there, but also being you, feeling your sensations, thinking your thoughts, experiencing your emotions. If you do this exploration about several different incidents, you will develop more ability to feel with and for each other – and thus develop more trust that you are understood.

Contacting the Feelings

Cutting off from emotions can lead to cutting off from physical sensation, too. Your goal is not only to get back in touch with your feelings and emotions, but also to find ways to cope with them when they are painful or negative – otherwise, your body will just shut down all sensation.

Begin by regularly being more aware of your body and how your emotions signal themselves to you – maybe a flush of pleasure along your stomach when you are looking forward to something, or a twinge in your back when you are irritated. Particularly, learn to recognize the sensations of positive emotion. Take time, maybe in bed each night, to review your positive sensations and emotions, particularly around sex.

Continue by being more open about what you feel with each other. Try telling your partner when you feel good about things, and feeling happy for her when she tells you her triumphs. Once you are at ease with this, try also expressing when you feel bad about things. To begin with, don't concentrate on when you feel bad about each other, just tell each other when you feel bad about work, home, the kids. But, instead of, as usual, simply letting off steam, try being very precise about what you are feeling. And, as you listen to your partner's negative feelings, don't cut her off or comfort her, just be interested in what she is describing to you. Eventually you will become more at ease with negative emotions, more able to realize that they are not frightening.

The next step, which may take a while, is to understand that it is OK to have negative feelings about each other, and to let them out. It is OK to fight and still love each other. You may be wary of doing this with the one you love because you fear this will drive her away – and such suppression of emotion can so easily lead to depression and consequent loss of desire.

If you really want to have a good sex life, then you need to learn to let the negatives out as early as possible, the first time you are aware of feeling them, whether this is in the kitchen or in bed. It has to be a fair fight – if one of you snipes and the other sulks, or one of you shouts so loud that the other can't get a word in edgeways, this technique won't work. What is needed is equal, energetic, enthusiastic bawling. It will burn itself up like a forest fire, and leave you feeling good, better, best – Supervirility!

Talking it Through

In general, you will probably be able to communicate with each other effectively, or you wouldn't have stayed together so long. First, though, check that you are still communicating in the way you did at the start of your partnership, or whether you have let things slide because you know each other so well. Remember that neither of you is a mind-reader, so a continual updating about what you feel and think is essential – otherwise, one day you will find you no longer know each other. And who wants to make love to an alienated stranger?

Secondly, even if you do still communicate well, hone your skills. When she speaks, listen to the underlying emotion as well as the words that are being said, or to the messages she gives from what you see as well as what you hear. Spend a day together not speaking, and see how far you can get just on the body language!

One particular communication issue in sex is asking and getting. RELATE's Marj Thoburn comments, 'Time after time, I make my clients smile when I tell them that they are trying to run a telepathic sexual relationship; they might hint at what they want, but they never actually say.'

You may be more comfortable love-making in silence, but you need a fairly constant flow of requests and feedback going from one to the other of you, otherwise, you simply fossilize into a narrower and narrower band of sexual action. Keep asking, on a minute-to-minute basis if you want to: 'Do that. Now there. Oh, that's lovely. No, do it harder, harder still, mmm.' Ask silently if you wish, with eye contact, touch, shifting movements and other such love-making codes.

As we point out in Chapter 9, however, being at ease with asking and getting doesn't mean to say that it is necessary for you or your partner to say yes to everything that is asked. If you want to say no, do so clearly, making sure your partner knows you still feel lovingly towards her, and perhaps offering an alternative that she wants. If you are refused, remembering that she is not refusing you, simply saying no to one of your suggestions. Also remember that pressurizing your partner will simply make her feel more threatened and so less sexual. To practise clean refusal, try saying no to each other once each day, and then talking through how that feels; it should begin to become less and less scary both to say and to hear. You could also both try going on assertiveness training courses designed to develop clear, honest communication skills.

> When it comes to talking things through in the general context of your relationship, over the next few weeks, take on board these guidelines: aim for equal power which leads to raised desire; never just blame; mention issues as soon as they arise; never say 'you always'; never walk out; never whinge; never threaten; never give in; never be afraid to negotiate; never go for the jugular; never talk more than you listen; always make it up by bedtime.

MAKING PROBLEM-SOLVING A SIGN OF LOVE

Whether in bed or out, reacting badly to each other's problems can trigger you into a spiral that can cause an anxiety-based block, such as erectile dysfunction (see page 92). Your goal should be to support each other effectively when problems arise, and not to panic.

In your relationship in general, learn to talk through any problems as they come up, concentrating on giving each other emotional support. Then see what you can agree on. If there is no point of agreement, then ask each other about your objections, and take them seriously; how can you meet them to find a solution that works for you both? For a relationship based on compromise or on one partner passively giving in is, in the long term, a relationship in which one of you will lose your desire. You have been warned!

If you hit a sexual block, either physical or emotional, while you are in bed, the first few seconds are often crucial. We have stressed over and over that the key here is not to carry on regardless, thinking that the other one will be disappointed, because you will get into a guilty anxiety spiral which will just make things worse next time round. First listen to one another as you explain why you are feeling emotional; at this point, the aim is actually not to solve the issue but to express and share without withholding the emotions that are arising. (If *after* some comfort and cuddles are offered, you decide to use oral or hand methods for one or both of you to orgasm, then this is fine.)

But once feelings have been shared and accepted by the other person, and once reassurance has been given, both in words and through cuddles, then set to, in a co-operative way, solving the problem together. Do you need help by oral sex? Does she need you to help by slowing down during intercourse? Do your tears indicate a need for counselling, or do they in fact show you are at last feeling secure enough to grieve for all the sad things that have happened between you in the past?

SETTING COMPELLING GOALS FOR YOURSELVES

What gives a relationship its zing is the thought that you have an exciting future together. This is what, at the start of a relationship, makes everything seem so bright and so wonderful; the reverse, the thought of a horrendous future, is what makes a bad relationship seem totally trapping.

We are assuming, if you are putting this much energy into enhancing your relationship, that your future together is secure; if not, then use your own resources and any outside help you need, to decide whether to stay together or not.

Then, talk more specifically about your sexuality. Begin by imagining that you are very old and that you have the sort of love life that people only dream about, still besotted with each other, having a better sex life day by day. Swap ideas with each other to put some detail on this broad picture, so that you are both clear about how good it could be. Then make a list of the things that you think you would need to do in order to create this sexual future for yourselves: get better at oral sex; break through your blocks on desire; give multiple orgasms. Choose three steps that you could take in the next month to work towards these changes: buy a vibrator; masturbate in front of each other at least once a week; tell each other a fantasy. Write these down and, at the end of the month, congratulate yourself on the actions you've completed. Plan three more for the next month.

CHECKING YOUR PROGRESS

The results of each piece of work you do may not come immediately. So don't worry if it takes a few weeks or even months for the benefits to filter through to your sex life. Particularly if you are working to re-establish desire that may have faded a long while ago, your bodies may be wary; it will take a while for them to trust that feeling sexual again is not going to cause problems, just as it did last time.

Equally, there may be a shake-down period, where you find yourselves more irritable or more angry with each other. In the same way as emptying the rubbish bin may mean a nasty smell, recontacting old emotions to clear them away may mean being reminded of them. Don't worry; this reaction will pass. Don't blame each other; you are both doing your best. If, in the long run, you find things are getting dramatically worse, then this may be the time to look for outside help. The chances are, however, that doing the explorations will make things dramatically better.

SUPERVIRILITY

OTHER OPTIONS
13

The fact has to be faced that your relationship is not the only place to fulfil your desire – and that, in order to be happy within your relationship, you may feel you need sexual input from elsewhere. This chapter aims to outline the possibilities of recreating your sexuality outside your current relationship.

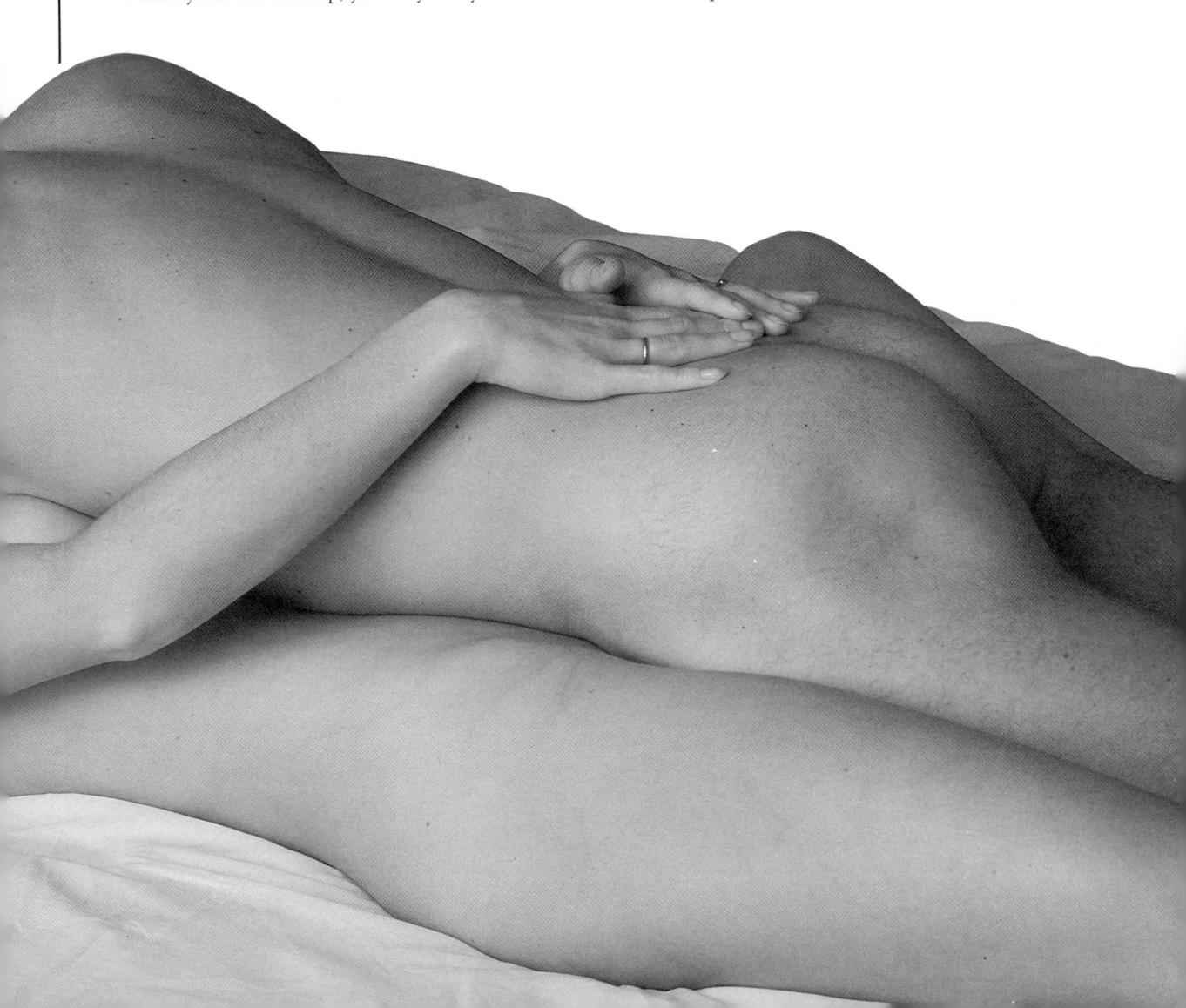

Erotica

Turning to books, magazines, films and videos of sex for erotic stimulation is part of most couples' repertoire; we explore more fully in Chapter 9 how you can best use it with your partner. If you are enjoying erotica without your partner, we would strongly advise you to try the end of the market that aims to pass on real knowledge as well as titillate, and the end of the market that tries to cater for women; they may seem less raunchy, but give you a far better idea of good technique and what women want. Of course, if you are using erotica as a substitute for, rather than an addition to, your partner, we do wonder whether you couldn't channel your energy into working to improve the relationship.

Where we as authors have real trouble with such erotica is where it is pornographic – in other words, either they suggest actions which are outside a loving range of sexual activity, or they perpetuate the mythical sex that we described in Chapter 7. This may be recreating the very sexual problem that underpins your dissatisfaction with your partner – the wish for idealized love-making. It certainly won't make your actual sex life any better and, if your partner finds out, it may be alienating, as much of this stuff is degrading.

Prostitutes

We personally can't condone the fact that many women are forced into prostitution unwillingly because of social conditions. That said, many prostitutes themselves believe that they are offering a public service and, for some men – who do not wish to threaten their sexless marriage by having an affair – going to a prostitute does seem like a sensible option.

There are very real dangers. Firstly, you may get a sexually transmitted disease, even AIDS. You may end up spending a lot of money. If your partner ever finds out, she may well be much more appalled by what she sees as sheer degradation than if you had screwed her best friend in the spare bedroom. And, of course, you are wrong if you seriously believe that spasmodic sex with an uninvolved professional will replace the all-round fulfilment of Supervirile sex. As with erotica, we would strongly advise you to use the money you are spending on your blow job to get some good couples' counselling!

If you do go to a prostitute, take precautions – always use a condom, even for oral sex. Take the emotional precaution of keeping well clear of anywhere you might be recognized by someone who knows your partner.

SUPERVIRILITY

HAVING AN AFFAIR

When Sue was researching for her recent book on affairs (*The Eternal Triangle*), she counted over thirty given reasons for people turning to sex outside their main relationship – and one of the chief of these was that sex with their original partner was unsatisfactory.

The classic justification calls on the Coolidge effect, from the infamous story of the American president whose wife was told by the owners of a chicken farm that the cockerel serviced the hens many times a day. 'Tell that to Mr Coolidge,' she said. On hearing it, Mr Coolidge quickly established that the cockerel's enthusiasm was raised by a large variety of hens. 'Tell that to Mrs Coolidge,' he retorted! Many men (and women) do believe that men are naturally polygamous and that it is only natural for them to seek variety. You can also see an affair as less threatening to a marriage than the possibility of divorce. You can view it as a boost to your ego, particularly if you are in the middle of a midlife crisis. You may feel it will take sexual pressure off your partner, or alternatively, act as a spur to renew interest.

Whatever reasons you have for sex outside your partnership, you need to realize that an affair will always rock the boat. Now, it could be that boat-rocking is exactly what is needed. You may want to break up an already-dead relationship. You may want to precipitate a crisis and so renew a nearly-dead relationship. You may know that the only way to get your partner's attention is to do something so awful that she has to listen to you. But once you start an affair, things will never be the same again.

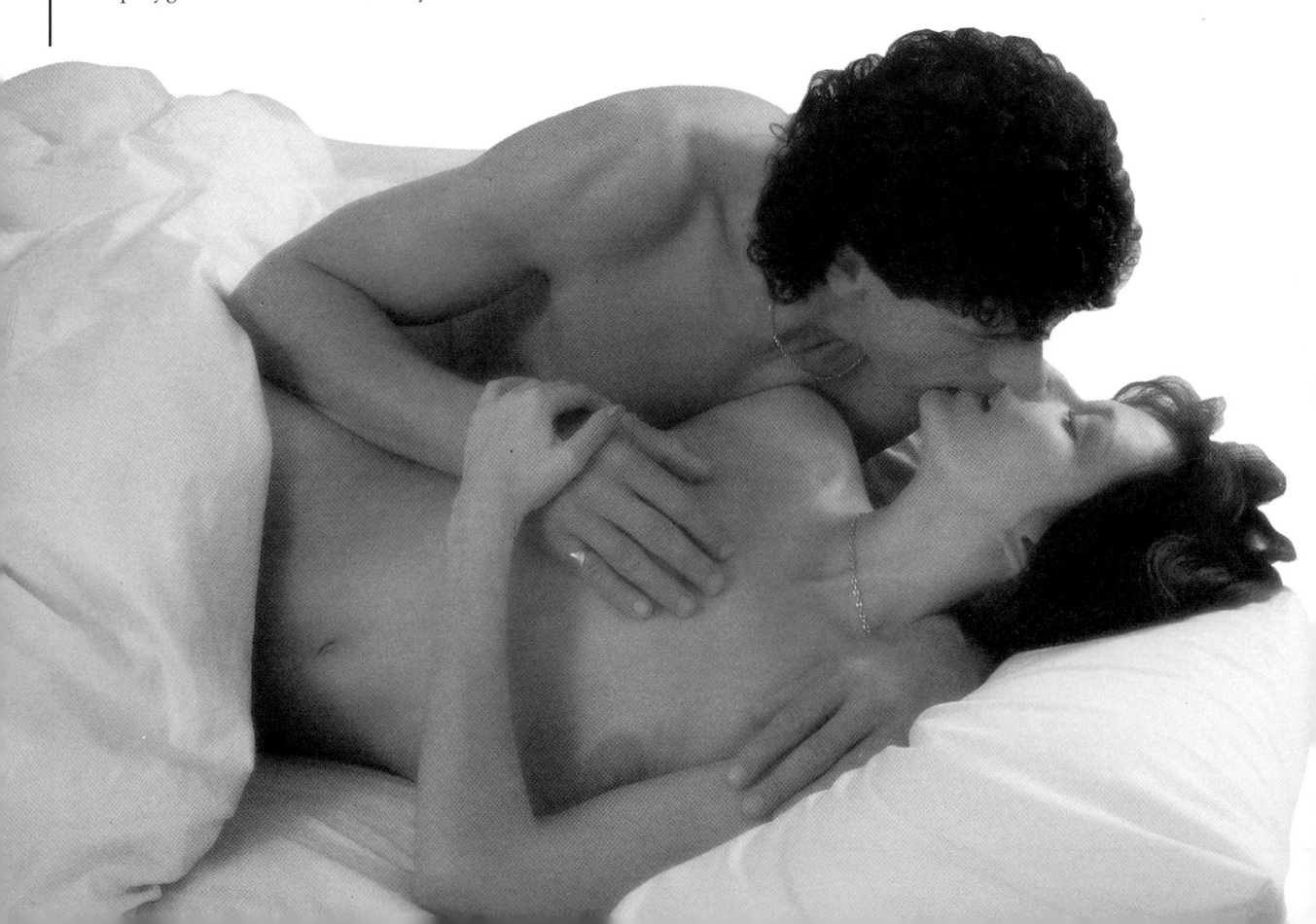

So before you begin, ask yourself why. If, in fact, you are looking for a replacement long-term partner, then be clear about this and finish one relationship before you start the next; this is kinder to everyone. Also bear in mind that the divorce rate for second marriages is higher than for first, and that if you change your partner without changing your attitude, you will end up with exactly the same problems all over again.

If you are simply looking for short-term sexual satisfaction which you are convinced is not possible within your current partnership, then first of all weigh up the possibility that, if discovered, you may lose your partner for good. If you feel the risk is worth it, then for heaven's sake choose a lover who is also in it for short-term pleasure, otherwise at best she will get hurt, and at worst all three of you will suffer. Look for her unconscious signals – not what she is saying she wants, but whether she is eyeing up baby clothes, or obviously undermining your present partner. If so, don't continue with a relationship that is so obviously a bad idea for your lover, even if it is a good idea for you.

What if, having walked the high wire quite successfully for a while, your partner finds out? You don't want to split up, she will have you back – but what about the future? You first have to re-establish trust within the relationship, and this will take all the skills we mention in Chapter 12 and a few more. Secondly, you have to face up to what will happen when things have stabilized again. Something has to change in your relationship and in your sex life, if you are not to find yourself repeating your mistake. Be reassured, however, that most couples who go to Relate with an affair-triggered crisis do stay together and are stronger for it.

Doing Without sex

Now here's something to make you think. Martin Cole, a leading sex therapist, argues that, for many people, desire for each other inevitably declines and that the closest partnerships are those most likely to suffer from this decline. He says, 'There is a built-in obsolescence to sexuality right from the start; sex can be inherently disruptive and creates unstable relationships.'

Dr Cole's approach is a shattering one, for he seems to be saying that you can have companionship and love, but you can't have sex as well. We hope he is wrong – but it could be that, faced with a stable and happy relationship that has lost all desire, you choose to accept his analysis and stick with your relationship. If you do, and if you feel as many men do that visiting prostitutes and having affairs would both be betrayals, then you are looking at the possibility of lifelong continence. This thought may frighten you.

The insight we would offer is this. Such a situation usually occurs because people believe that both of them have to agree on a course of action in order to change the situation. This is just not true. You do not need your partner to agree to become more sexual, or to have sex with you, or to agree to change, or to go to counselling, in order for the relationship to alter. If you yourself go for counselling, this will automatically shift the emotional balance. It may make you more accepting of your partner's asexuality. It may make you more at ease with having an affair. It may make you decide to end the relationship and start another, more sexual one. Or it may make you accept the thought of continence for the rest of your life, happy to do that because your relationship is so valuable. Do try it; seek to make some sort of change yourself, without putting pressure on your partner; something will alter, and it will certainly be for the better.

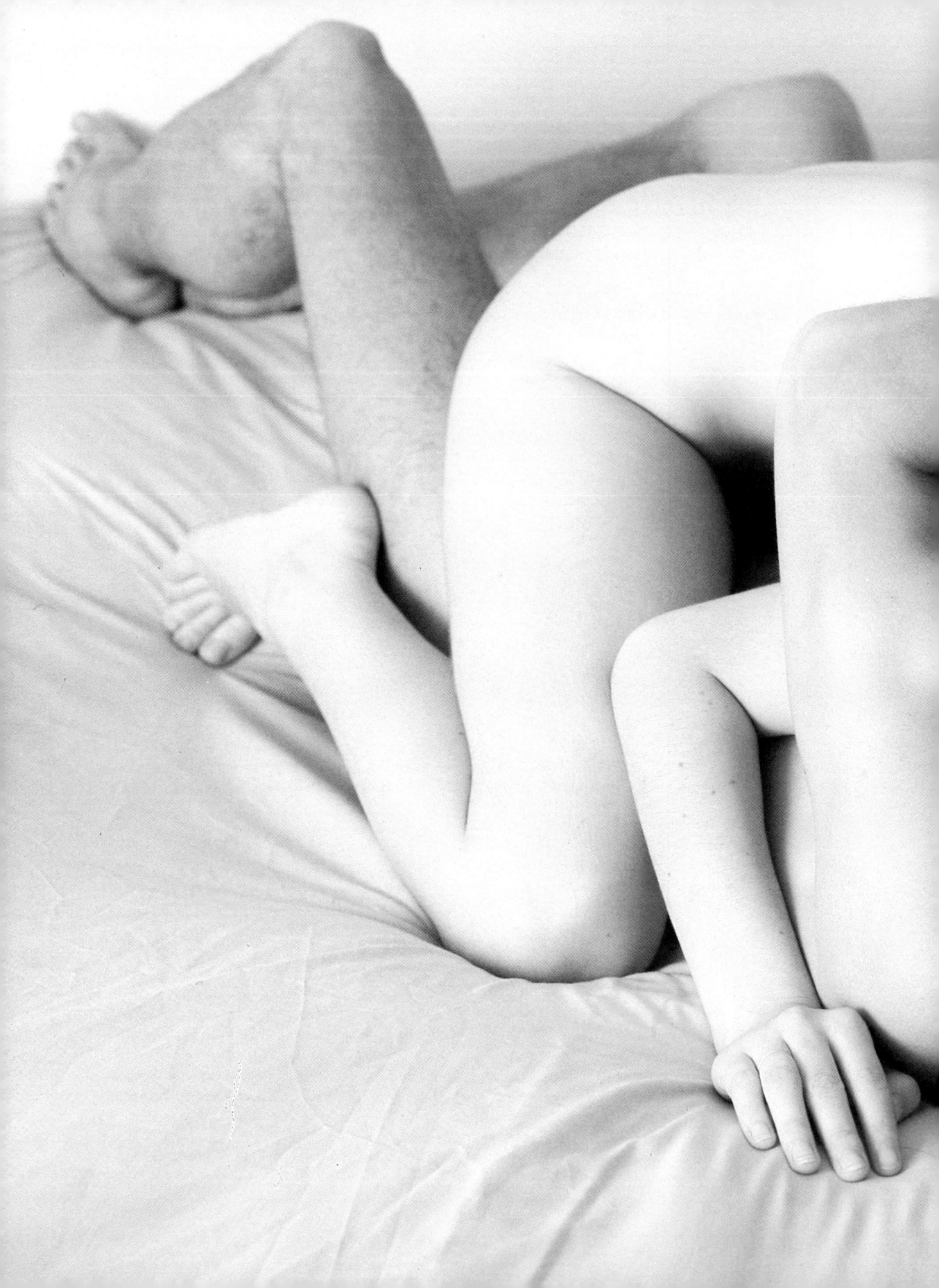

PART IV
SEXUAL SUPERVIRILITY

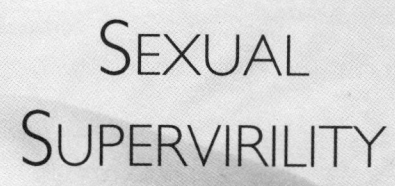

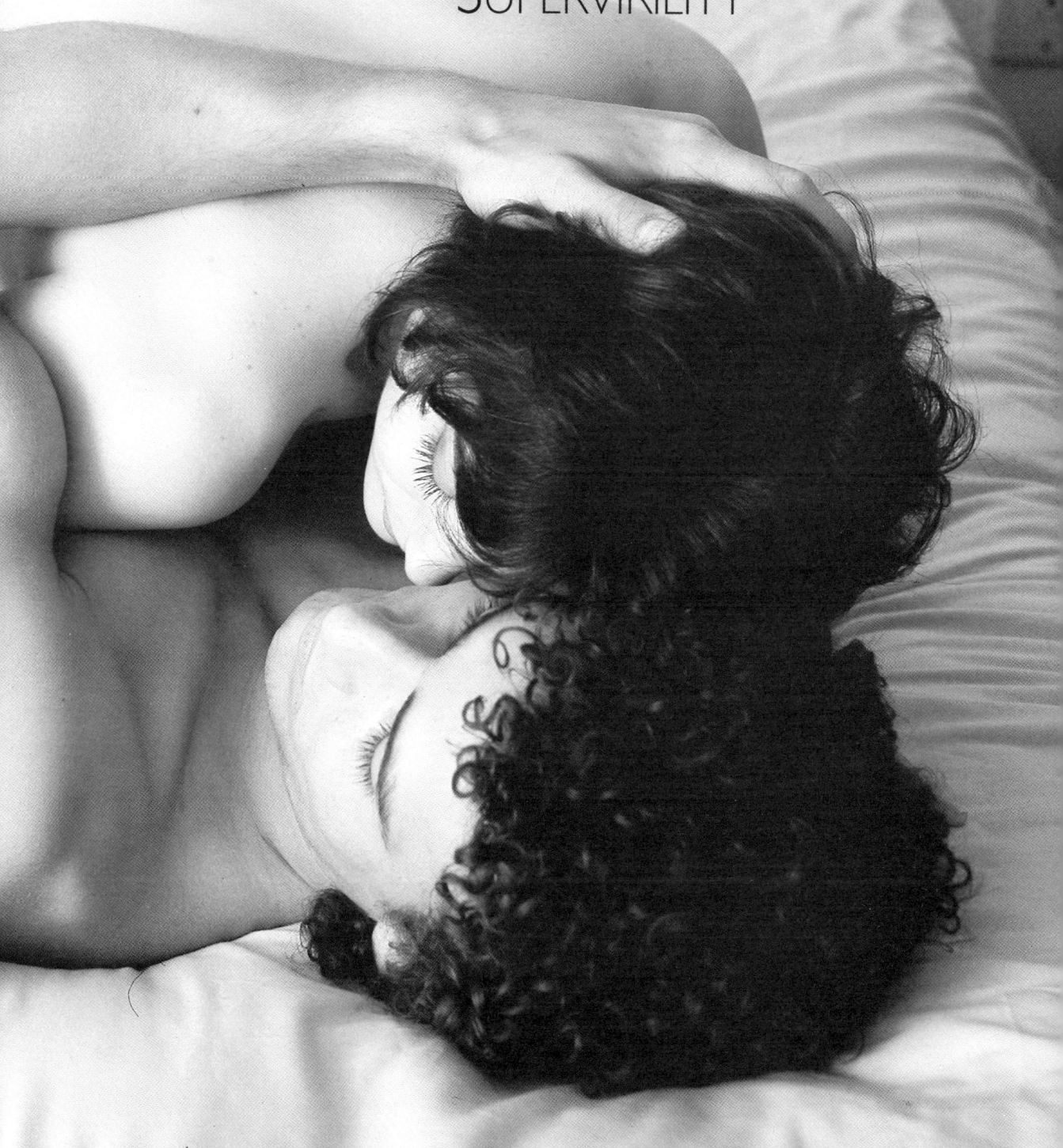

Her Body, Her Sexuality

For far too many of us, it is sexual technique that needs the attention if we are to gain Supervirility. Sex tends to be something we never learn and are never taught. By the time we find the partner with whom we can take the time to learn, perhaps we feel embarrassed to stop and wonder; we think we should know, and don't like to ask. Then, we find it difficult to adapt our technique to suit the passing of time, and we no longer know just how to combine experience and skill to fit our changing needs.

This section of the book outlines, step-by-step, ways in which men can re-learn about sex. More than that, it offers a sequence of sexual explorations which will allow you and your partner together to contact your arousal potential and then expand it through to Supervirility.

Before you begin, however, you need to know just how your partner's body works, what the key erotic areas for her are, just how she gets aroused and moves towards orgasm. Knowing this is as vital to your fulfilling your sexual potential as is knowing about yourself and your own arousal patterns. If your partner feels able to accompany this brief physical description by a practical reminder of what her intimate parts looks like, then all the better; but if that's not appropriate, simply remember what we are saying here until the next time you have a chance to look closely at your partner's body.

Her Body

How is your partner's body like yours? The skeleton, the nerves, the blood and the bone are similar. She may be smaller, slimmer, less muscular than you – but the essential inner workings of sensing erotic stimuli, carrying the message to the brain and using hormones to arouse are all the same.

A much wider area of your partner's skin than yours is erotically sensitive; her erogenous zones can cover her entire body, her sensitivity is likely to be greater. Her breasts are perhaps sensitive all over, perhaps only on the aureola and nipple, perhaps not at all. Your partner's genitals, unlike yours, are hidden, tucked away between her legs.

The outer and inner lips of her genitals open to reveal her clitoris and vagina. The clitoris, a miniature penis with shaft, glans and hood, is almost certainly her most sensitive part. The entrance to the vagina, behind the clitoris and in front of her anal passage, leads to the cervix, the entrance to her womb; it is the vagina that you penetrate during intercourse, and it is the cervix through which sperm travel if you ejaculate freely inside your partner. Some experts say that just inside the vagina on the wall nearest the clitoris, there is a particularly sensitive 'G'-spot that can bring great arousal at orgasm; there is an equally sensitive spot between vagina and rectum, and both of these points are worthwhile exploring during sex.

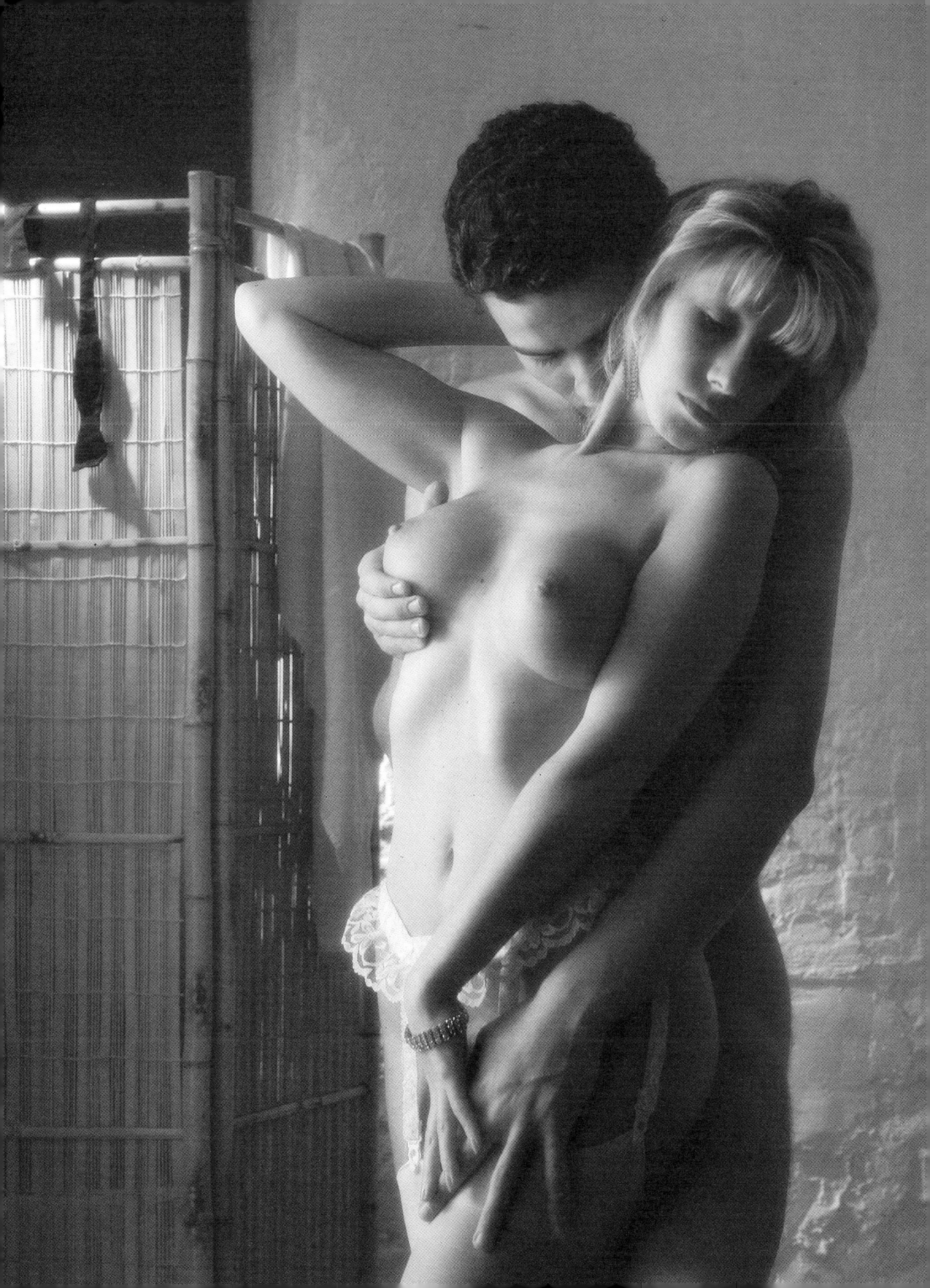

Her Arousal

What happens for your partner during arousal parallels what happens for you. Like you, during love-making, her body will respond with all the classic signs of arousal: rising heart rate, breathing and blood pressure, tensed muscles, enlarged pupils and increased sensitivity. If her excitement rises, she too will hit the plateau phase, where her body is ready to tip over into orgasm. Her breasts may enlarge and her nipples erect. She may have a sex flush on chest and tummy. Her vagina, which may flood with moisture as she gets excited, will also balloon out to allow penetration. Though only the entrance to the vagina is really sensitive, its entire length will lubricate. Her clitoris will engorge with blood as she becomes more and more aroused, the hood easing back from its sensitive tip.

When she does tip over into orgasm, your partner's rhythm coincides with yours, with contractions of one every 0.8 seconds. But she can have many different kinds of orgasm: one which begins in her clitoris; one which is felt mainly in her vagina; a total body orgasm where every muscle is involved; a quiet sigh or shudder; a series of ascending peaks in multiple orgasm.

Like you, her body needs to rest once she has come; but for a much shorter time, sometimes only seconds. Then the rise can begin again, and she can continue to yet another peak.

You may like to remember, as you review this description, all the times when you have seen your partner aroused, recalling just what her excitement looks like, and how she reacts when she is pleasured. What are her signs of enjoyment? How can you tell when she is rising up the arousal scale? Does she have signals to tell you if she is coming? How can you tell when she is ready to begin again?

Her Blocks

Like you, your partner may be experiencing sexual blocks. And, although this is not a book aimed specifically at women's issues, any blocks she may have will, of course, affect you.

She may, for example, be suffering from the effects of getting older. Child-bearing may have shifted her body's sexual response, taking the urgency away and making sex something that she is simply not motivated to do. Equally, your partner's body in general, and her sexual parts in particular, may have changed with the menopause, diminishing desire and including the possibility of vaginal dryness and discomfort on penetration.

It could be, too, that specifically your partner is non-orgasmic. We as authors have a dual attitude to this. On the one hand, we believe that it is unhelpful to insist that every woman must have an orgasm, just as it is unhelpful to insist that every man must have an erection; so if your partner is non-orgasmic and genuinely happy with that situation, then we would strongly recommend that you back her in her decision. Nevertheless, we also believe that every woman has a right to orgasm, and that if she cannot come and wants to, then she needs every possible form of support.

Certainly, the explorations we suggest later in this part will make an orgasm for your partner much more likely. The gentle, sensuous touching, the emphasis on oral and hand stimulation, the experimentation with intercourse position, will all give her the opportunity to get what pleases her. Crucially, taking an active role in giving and receiving pleasure will help her to find out what she wants and go for that. You may also want to support your partner in her own programme of learning how to touch herself, how to reach orgasm on her own, and then how to teach you what she has learned about her arousal process. Appendix B recommends some useful organizations for further support.

How the Mismatch Works

Although male and female responses are similar, there may be, as we mentioned in Chapter 10, a basic mismatch here for many couples, which has to be reconciled before you can begin to make sex as good as it can be. You and your partner may, of course, not have this mismatch – or may already know about it and have found a solution between you. Yet, it is worthwhile for you to explore it again – misunderstanding it is one of the key ways that mutual satisfaction gets blocked.

The first manifestation of mismatch is that women's patterns of arousal may differ from those of men. Women may need prolonged foreplay to become aroused; they may need copious arousal to make penetration pleasurable. Women can tend to take far longer than men to reach their peak – so while he is coming for the first time, she may be barely aroused. Conversely, while he then needs time to recover, she wants to keep going – and can do so through many hours of arousal, excitement and repeated orgasm. Naturally, as we are all different, some women get aroused and come very quickly, particularly at the start of a relationship; but many don't.

The second manifestation of the issue is that, for her, penetration may be less likely to lead to orgasm, however long it lasts. Of course, every woman is different; many do get a great deal out of penetration. But she may need her clitoris touched by hand or mouth; she may need a position of intercourse that stimulates her clitoris; she may need two or three manual orgasms before the arousal begins to reach her vagina. Critically, however aroused she becomes, she may need clitoral stimulation all the way up to her climax, not simply to start her off. So once the 'foreplay' stage – which for men may seem a rather boring preliminary – is over, the effect of penetration for her may actually be anti-climactic. Imagine if someone making love to you expected you to come while they were simply stroking your balls!

All the above is not a new theory – or a product of women's lib. Many non-Western love traditions say that no woman can reach orgasm without oral sex or very careful positioning of bodies. It is not a case of immaturity or frigidity, as doctors, biologists and even eminent sex therapists such as Masters and Johnson have claimed. It is often simply a case of physiology!

If you have previously been unaware of these mismatches, you may find this explanation hard to understand or to accept. You may wonder whether it is possible for a man and a woman to make love successfully; if he has to hold back for ages for her, or she cannot come with penetration, how on earth are they to manage mutual sexuality?

The Good News

The answer to these questions is twofold. First, mutual sexuality is a total package. Perhaps up to now, in Western society at least, the emphasis has been on performance, erection and penetration. But other civilizations have known for centuries that this is just one option, and that love-making can follow many different routes to orgasm. Love-making is about sight, sound, smell, taste, touch, licking, fondling, moving, lying still and pushing yourselves to higher and higher peaks of pleasure – some of which have to do with erection and some of which do not, some of which have to do with putting your penis in her vagina, and some of which do not.

Secondly, what appears in most Western erotica, films, books and magazines is kindergarden sex. What we are aiming at, in Supervirility, is graduate sex, with options including erection and penetration, but with other options that go far beyond that. And these options transcend the mismatches that we have just outlined. She may learn to come with penetration, by using added positions and stimulation that allow her to orgasm. You may learn to enjoy sensuality throughout your body which does not depend on erection or penetration. You may both learn to time your love-making so that you drift in the plateau phase while she takes her first orgasm, then her second, and you finally climax together on her third.

There is more good news. This graduate sex, this Supervirility, is most possible for men who are older. Supervirility is not at its peak at seventeen, whatever the biological evidence. With the passage of time, you become more and more able to be Supervirile.

How does this happen? To begin with, all these options we've just described depend on experience. They need to be learned slowly, integrating them into our relationship within a mature framework of love, commitment and sexual knowledge. Needless to say, the possibility of all this increases year by year.

Also, many of these advanced techniques actually depend on the particular sexual patterns of a man past his youthful lust. For, as time passes, he is more and more able to slow down his reactions and delay his ejaculation. While men are panicking because they can no longer come in three minutes, women are heaving a sigh of relief that their men are now capable of prolonged love-making! And once these advanced techniques have been mastered, men too can be enjoying the exquisite pleasure of the plateau phase before orgasm, which may only now, for the first time, be really possible for them.

And, as instant automatic erection becomes less likely for a man as time passes, so he becomes more able to opt for other things, for his partner and for himself. He may start to develop finger and tongue technique, seeing them now not as optional foreplay, but as essentials in his repertoire. He may start to be able to accept greater stimulation on his penis, more pleasuring, more fantasy, more lubrication – in fact, more of everything that can give him extended pleasure, and which before, his instant erection simply couldn't handle. With age, a man may also begin to accept that his partner can have the kind of active role in stimulation and love-making that is essential to advanced love-making.

Finally, these techniques, which bring together male and female sexual cycles and allow women to reach orgasm, can often largely bypass any seeming 'problems' that men reach as life goes on. By opening out sexuality from concentrating on erection-penetration, these techniques avoid boredom, as well as reducing performance anxiety. By making it essential that both woman and man are equally involved in love-making, each asking for and getting what they really want, these techniques give the co-operative stimulation that may be necessary for the man to get it up – and for the woman to come. By creating a sex act that actually depends on prolonging pleasure and not going for quick release, these techniques make the whole of love-making more enjoyable – and so remove the fear of declining sexuality that may haunt us as we leave our youth.

COMPARING NOTES

To start integrating all these thoughts and suggestions, you may need time to think. This exploration may help. To attempt it, you need to have sound trust between you and your partner, and to feel secure in each other's love.

Sit together, facing each other, perhaps on the bed, perhaps naked. Take it in turns to answer these questions, one at a time. Ask all the questions, even if you have already discussed some of them earlier in your relationship. While you are listening to the answers, hold back interruptions, reassurances or explanations. Once your partner has finished talking, you can ask further questions – but resist the temptation to get defensive or explanatory (Oh, the reason I don't do that is... Oh, but you always said...). This is an information-exchange session, not a discussion. Add in hugs, cuddles – or practical demonstrations – if you need to. If the session turns to love-making, that's fine!

1. In general, what do you like best about the way we make love now?

2. What is particularly good about the foreplay we have? Tell me three ways it could be better.

3. (*Her asking, him answering*) When we come to your erection, tell me three ways we could together support you more to get the erection you want.

4. What is good about the way we masturbate each other? By hand? By mouth? Tell me three ways that could be better.

5. (*Him asking, her answering*) When we come to penetration, is it usually too early, too late, or just about right for you? Tell me three ways that we could make penetration and intercourse better for you.

6. (*Him asking, her answering*) In general, is penetration a way that you can achieve orgasm? If not, do you want to? Have you achieved orgasm through penetration within the last ten times we have made love? If so, what did we do to make that happen? If not, tell me three things we could do to make that happen or three ways we could help you to get orgasms through masturbation, if that is what you'd prefer?

7. (*Her asking, him answering*) Tell me three things we could do to help you come less quickly, more quickly.

8. Tell me three things we could do to help you get an even better orgasm.

9. Tell me three things we could do to make the time after love-making even more satisfying for you.

This exploration is essential to the whole concept of fulfilled love-making; so don't think of it as a once-and-for-all thing. Repeat it regularly, every few months or so, to update each other constantly on your desires.

SUPERVIRILITY

First Moves

15

The very first hint of love-making will come from your mind rather than your body. Whether or not you are aware of it, the thought of how good it would be to make love comes into your awareness. So hang on to this mental arousal and use your own mind to enhance your desire.

At some point, you will need to know that your partner is also preparing for sex. By this time in your relationship, whether you know it or not, you will probably have developed personal codes, a particular glance or intonation, a hug that turns into something else. Perhaps you have prolonged eye contact, a slight shift in the way you smell to each other, a slight difference in the way you move.

What if your partner is genuinely not willing? We personally think that, if so, you should find some other way to bring yourself pleasure – although, of course, if your partner consistently pulls back from love-making when you want it, you need to challenge what is happening.

How could you, also, encourage your partner to make the first move herself? First, remind her that you'd love it if she jumped you. Secondly, react positively if she does.

And if you both decide to watch TV? That's fine; the golden rule of good sex is never to do anything you don't really want to do. You have learned a valuable lesson; that you can say no and still love each other. Next time will be even better.

Setting the Scene

Having begun to make love, albeit still in your thoughts, set the scene. There is a certain delight in making love somewhere unusual and risky; in the back of a car, in the woods, across the dining-room table. For most of us, though, sex means bed. Make sure that it is comfortable; beds for couples should be bought with an eye to enough width for stretching across, enough height to allow either of you to sit on or kneel by it while pleasuring or being pleasured, and enough firmness to allow good purchase when moving into different positions. We find that a duvet gives a light covering that moves as you do – and remember that pillows are fine for sleeping, but may simply get in the way during love-making, although one or two available for popping under buttocks or backs may make all the difference for pleasure or comfort.

Make sure all your senses are pleased, by a comfortable setting that looks good and is sufficiently dimly lit; music is a good background and has the added advantage of cutting out any internal mental conversation about how well (or badly) you are doing. It also helps you to concentrate on what is happening in the here and now rather than spectatoring.

Find ways to involve the often-forgotten senses smell and taste. Alert your body to what is to follow by incense, fresh flowers and wonderful-tasting food and drink – particularly the sort you can eat in bed and feed to each other (though serve nothing crumbly, or the bits will get everywhere!)

Finally, explore touching. Well before clothes come off, you should be making contact, holding hands, stroking each other's face, rubbing feet. What keeps a couple together, far more than orgasms, is cuddles, the warmth, softness and total reassurance of your bodies touching along their entire length. Learn how to hug and you will learn how to love.

Finally, one particular ritual that we personally reckon should be part of every couple's scene-setting, is to check out contraception. Perhaps the whole topic is not a concern for you any more, because of sterilization, or because your partner is through the change of life. But if contraception is still a live issue, then once in a while check out with each other whether you are both still happy with the options you are taking. And remember that, whatever your birth control needs, some health professionals are currently recommending using a condom, because of the protection it gives you against STDs.

Aphrodisiacs – or Not?

The argument rages. Are there aphrodisiacs or are there not? When researching this book, we read several medical textbooks which stated decisively (and defensively) that there were absolutely no ways of rekindling sexual desire. Most sex manuals too assured us that the only aphrodisiac was real love.

Historically the endless list of exotic aphrodisiacs, such as powdered lion's penis and rhinoceros horn, mandrake root and turtles' eggs, seems never to have been reliable enough to be consistently recommended. Some, like Spanish fly made from beetles ground into powder, are actually dangerous and can fatally irritate internal organs. Nowadays some recreational drugs have the street reputation of increasing sexual pleasure, but while amyl nitrate, cocaine and hallucinogens are said to intensify sensation in the short term, they seem to have nasty side-effects, both medically and in terms of their illegality.

Alcohol in tiny doses has been proved to lower inhibition as well as raising sensory awareness (clink glasses with your lover to make a drink of wine involve five senses, not just four), though as the infamous quote in *Macbeth* comments, 'Alcohol provokes the desire but takes away the performance' (Act 2, sc 3, 134).

What about food? Recent research has shown that chocolate, traditionally the favourite gift from a man to a woman, contains phenylethylamine, which when found in the brain produces all the emotions and actions of infatuation and love – energy, elation, euphoria. So when you and your partner eat chocolates together, you are enhancing your natural feeling for each other by the substances you eat.

Yohimbine, a herbal remedy found in the bark of the yohimbe tree, has a reputation for increasing potency. This has not been proved; research studies which seem to show promising results are based on a prescription drug very different from the products sold over the counter. However, there is a large-scale clinical trial currently being run in Britain, and in time this will give a clearer picture.

Among herbs, the ancient Chinese remedy ginseng has recently enjoyed a reputation for stimulating sex drive, and modern research is still being carried out in China on its effects. Catuaba bark and guarana capsules, both from the Amazon rainforests, are possible aphrodisiacs.

Turning to spices, many have been recommended down through the ages: cayenne pepper, cinnamon, saffron. Nutmeg is said to delay ejaculation, though it causes severe hangover if taken in too-large doses. Ginger, an ancient Eastern aphrodisiac, is currently recommended as a cure for impotence by at least one chain of high street healthfood shops. It can be eaten or rubbed into the penis to cause erotic tingling during oral sex or intercourse; a mixture of preserved ginger and honey can be smeared over the penis and left for your partner to lick off at her leisure, or you can enter her and share the hot sensations.

Erotic Thoughts

Use your thoughts to build the atmosphere and to enhance your sensations. Allow your thoughts to wander; don't limit yourself to the here-and-now, but start exploring all kinds of options in your mind as a prelude to love-making. Don't feel guilty at what you imagine, and don't worry if as the fantasy develops it begins to include people other than your partner. This is not a sign of fading love, but of being free to explore possibilities. Most people, if given the chance to put their fantasy into reality, would actually run a mile!

So where would you like to be, with whom, when and in which situation? Extend your repertoire as far as you like, and allow your mind to take you places you could never be in real life.

If you feel at a loss, and want a starting point, remember that the Japanese used what they call 'pillow books', which contain erotic drawings of different positions, not only for reference *in situ*, but also to arouse mentally. The Western equivalent, erotica (distinguished from pornography by the fact that it offers a positive, sensuous view of sex), is also useful to start you thinking and to provide a starting point for the words. See Appendix C for some recommended reading.

The opposite of erotic fantasies are the negative or spectator-like thoughts that often intrude (Am I doing it right? I'll never make it), at this stage or later in love-making. Remember that you do have a choice of whether to think them or not. Don't tensely try to banish them – they'll just cling on harder; instead, replace them with positive thoughts about the good things you are enjoying (I'm doing fine... we can have oral sex if I don't make it).

At the same time, fully relax your body to make the blocks disappear. Use the 'tense–relax' exercise we suggest in Chapter 2, or, during love-making, take a deep, long breath. Breathe in not simply from your chest, but from the top of your head to the tips of your toes. Make it a long movement that involves the whole of you, and uses your lungs, chest and abdomen, so that you are aware of it throughout your entire body. As you breathe out air involve your whole body and feel yourself relax deeply. As you breathe in and out again, make this next breath longer, more relaxing than the previous one. Breathe a third, even longer breath, and relax even more deeply as you breathe out. This Eastern technique for relaxing into your breathing also helps keep erections firm and extends love-making as long as possible.

SOUNDS AND WORDS

You will almost certainly have non-verbal ways of expressing your thoughts to one another – little murmurs, grunts, movements and shifts, codes that tell each other what you are thinking and feeling. A good lover is aware of these, and keeps refining them, making sure that they are kept alive and changing by use. Such codes are not only a superb way of communication, but also a way of strengthening your relationship.

Equally, talking is often a forgotten part of sexuality. Tell her how wonderful she is, particularly what you like about her body and her sexuality – and make sure that the words continue as you become more and more aroused.

So become aware of words that you feel able to use with each other, to talk about what you are doing. Take time, perhaps as part of loveplay, to explore the words you most like to use and to check out that they are ones she is also comfortable with. Below are some starters. Alongside each, write several of the words you know that refer to these things. Then underline or simply tell your partner which are your favourites, and which you don't like to use. When she has completed her list, learn from that, too.

Use these words, even right at the start of love-making, to describe what you are going to do to each other, or what you want your partner to do to you. Keep communicating what you want – it turns sex into a constantly improving mutual dynamic.

Even without touching, words can inflame – try finding one phrase that arouses you both and try saying it over and over in turn, keeping eye contact and letting the touching develop from this.

Equally, there are few things more erotic than being aroused to the accompaniment of your own or your partner's whispered voice describing in graphic detail all the erotic fantasy elements you most enjoy. Go for the small detail, the way things look and sound, smell and taste, feel and respond. The story does not need to have a beginning or an end, and it often works better if you tell it in the first person. To start, try the phrases 'Do you know what I'm imagining happening now? Do you know what I'd be doing to you if...' or 'Tell me what you're imagining happening now...' 'What do you imagine me doing to you if we were...'

Take turns to weave a story – and then challenge each other to imagine something even more fantastic next time.

penis	giving oral sex to you	penetration
testicles	giving hand masturbation to you	intercourse
vagina	giving oral sex to her	the point of no return
clitoris	giving hand masturbation to her	orgasm

SENSUAL TOUCHING

16

To fully enjoy sex, extend your horizons to include touching – well before the first hint of erection occurs. The temptation may be to see sensual touching as being mere foreplay, dispensable as a relationship develops. We personally are convinced that true Supervirility means extending sensuous touching so that it runs throughout every aspect of love-making. This is not to say that there is no place for a straight in-and-out quickie – but such rushes of lust are only really possible in a long-term relationship if you keep arousal high by indulging constantly in sensuality.

For sensual touching is important to our sanity and our relationships. Human beings suffer from a general tactile starvation; as adults, we have few opportunities for physical contact, without which, as babies, we can get seriously ill. And regular contact on a sensory level is essential for the development of a growing relationship – if not, we will literally drift apart. Equally, prolonged non-erectile contact makes for better sex in the end. It means that she is more aroused. It means that you feel less pressured to perform. It means that you are both given the chance to learn more about each other, well before the demands of sexuality begin.

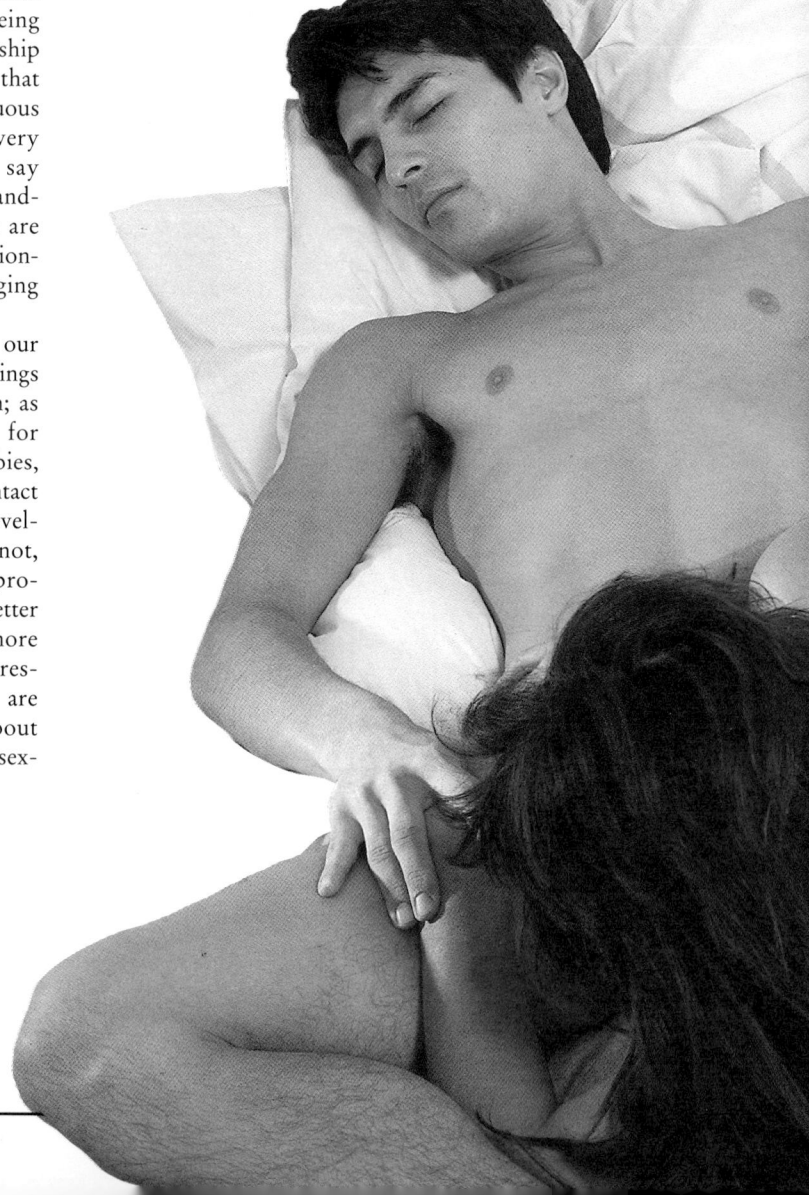

SENSUAL TOUCHING

UNDRESSING AND AFTER

All too often, used to undressing efficiently at night in order to sleep, you forget the other options. For long, slow love-making, remember that undressing each other, with long, slow kisses in between, is incredibly arousing. Try a hurried scrabble to get clothes off as quickly as possible; or leaving most of your clothes on and simply baring the essential bits. Try it with your eyes closed, going only by touch – and accept the burst of giggles that will come if you get stuck with her bra fastenings. Or, keep your eyes wide open and tell her lovingly how you feel about each part of her body when it emerges.

Once naked, what about taking a bath or shower together – or a sauna or jacuzzi if from there it is only a step to the bedroom? Hot water is a wonderful relaxant; you can add different smells, along with bubbles and soothing oils. Candles in the bathroom can replace the harshness of overhead lighting, and a glass of cold white wine each will create a wonderful interplay with the warmth of the water. Experiment, too, with the shower attachment which, underwater, can cause wonderful rippling effects against skin. She may leap ahead if it is lightly used on her clitoris, and be ready for orgasm long before you are!

Once out of the bath, try a relaxing massage. Make sure the room is warm, and lie the massage receiver on the bed or even floor, padded with a blanket or cushions that won't ruin if you get oil on them. Massage lotion such as you can buy at the Body Shop, is often beautifully scented and designed so that it stays on the surface of the skin and lubricates the movement of your hands; pour it into a bowl so you can reach it easily while massaging. The massage giver should wash their hands and remove jewellery beforehand.

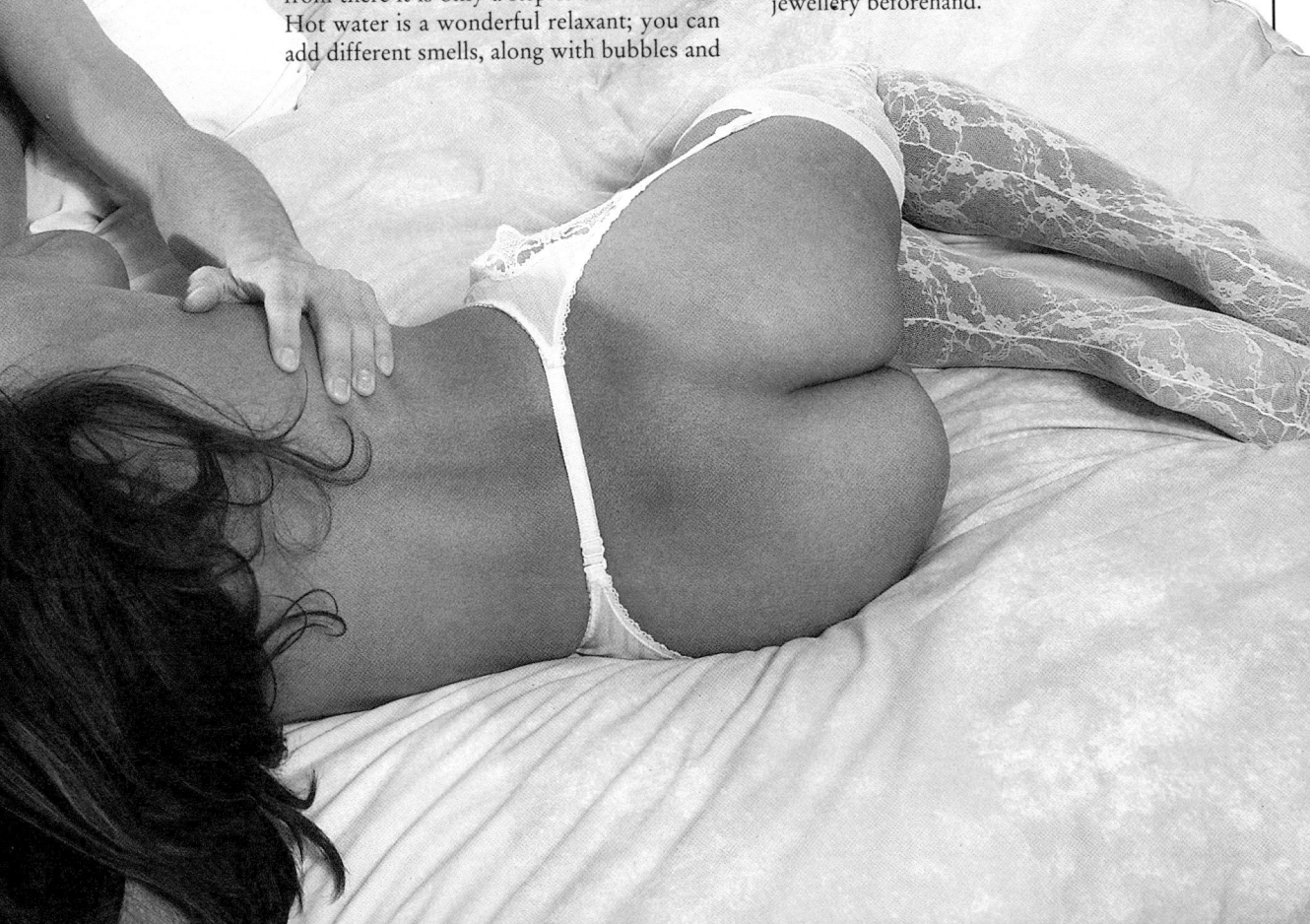

Massage Hints

Although there are many books giving detailed instructions about giving massage, doing it intuitively often works just as well if you follow these simple instructions.

- Keep clear of anywhere vulnerable, such as infected skin, scars, varicose veins or the abdomen if she is pregnant.

- Keep clear of the spine (the muscles on either side of the spine, on the other hand, often love a little pressure).

- Avoid 'sound and fury'; the best massage is quiet, slow and firm: most beginners either go too quickly or too lightly. Explore skin and muscle, at first encouraging your partner to tell you what feels best, then once you have learnt, letting her relax and silently enjoy being explored.

- Never stop touching your partner during a massage; if you lean over for extra oil, keep one hand in contact or she is likely to feel abandoned as she wonders where your hand has gone.

- Keep massage balanced on both sides. If you massage one arm, do the other one. Use both hands, one on each side of her back. Both hands massaging simultaneously in the same way on opposite sides of the body is wonderful.

- If you see or feel a flinch or a sudden tension, or hear a noise that indicates tension or pain, change what you are doing and go more slowly and gently.

- If you see or feel a softening or a melting, or hear breath or sound that indicates comfort and relaxation, keep doing what you are doing – for a long time!

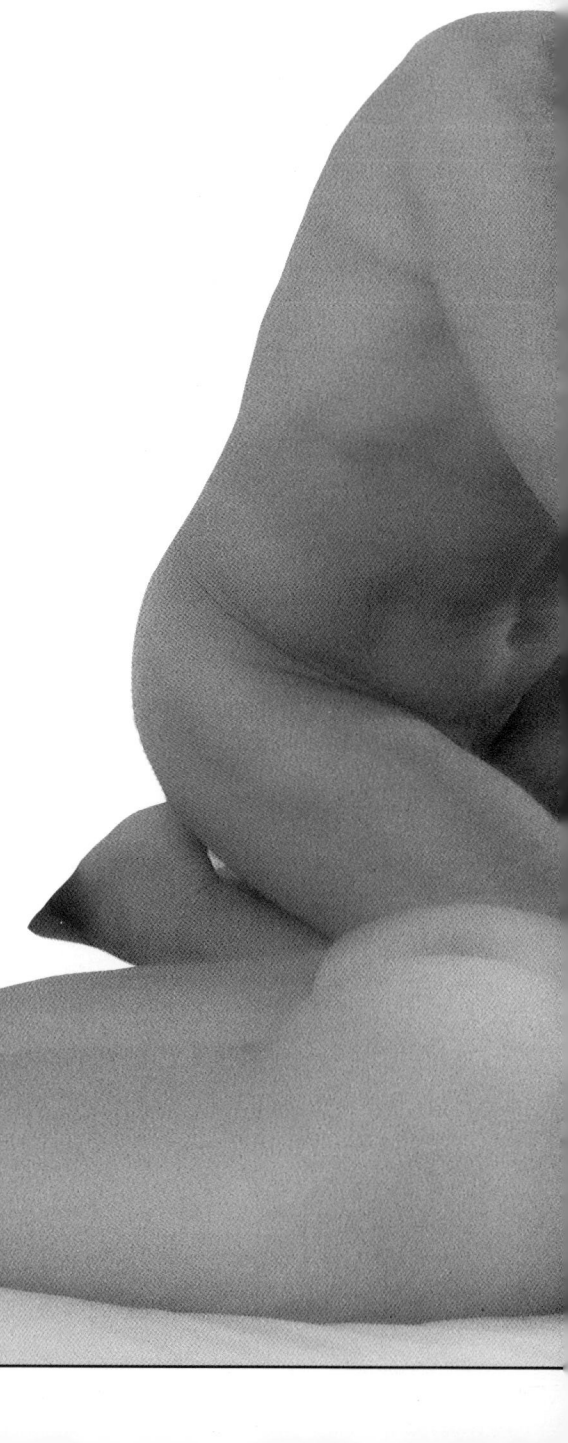

— SENSUAL TOUCHING —

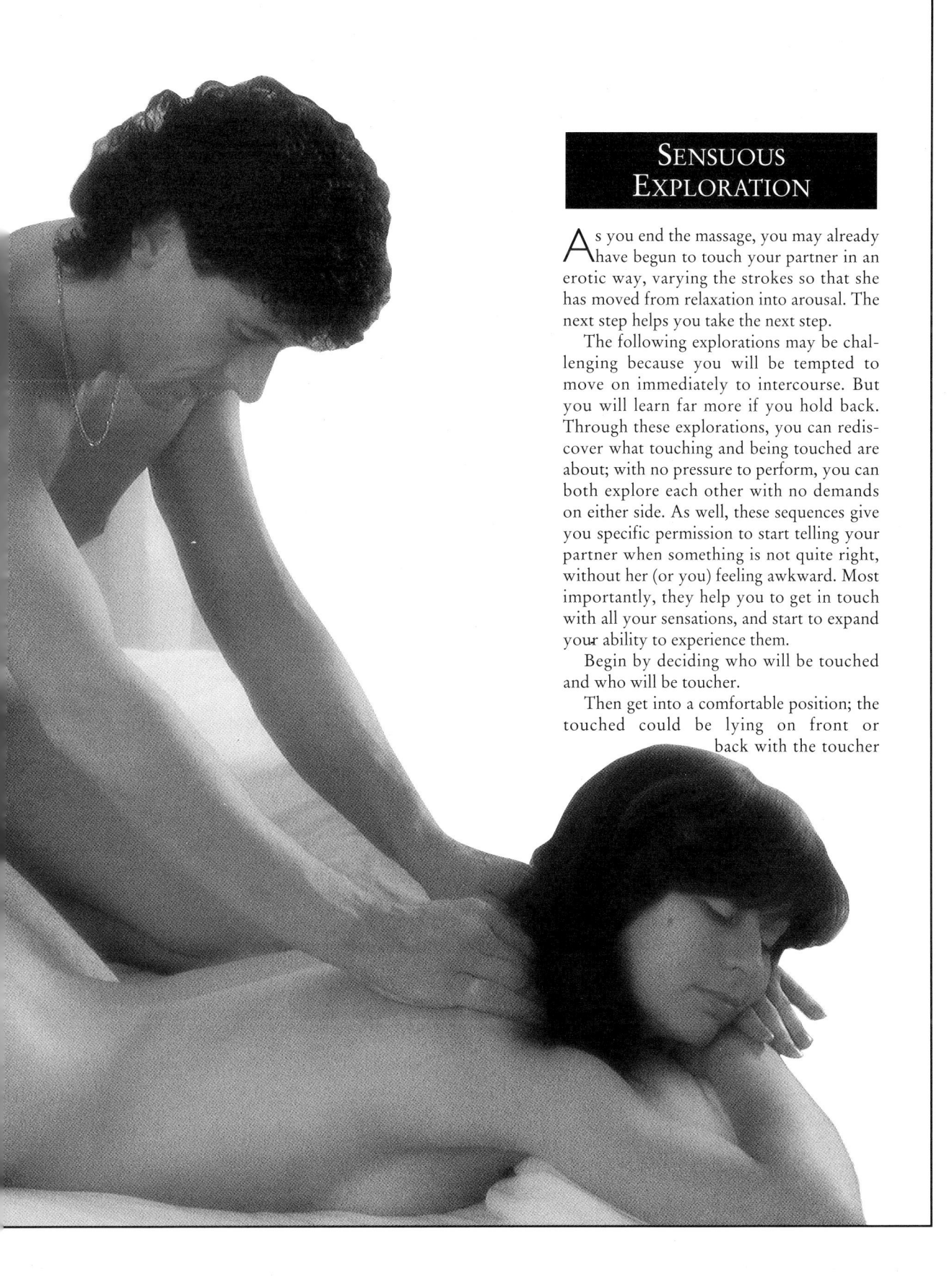

SENSUOUS EXPLORATION

As you end the massage, you may already have begun to touch your partner in an erotic way, varying the strokes so that she has moved from relaxation into arousal. The next step helps you take the next step.

The following explorations may be challenging because you will be tempted to move on immediately to intercourse. But you will learn far more if you hold back. Through these explorations, you can rediscover what touching and being touched are about; with no pressure to perform, you can both explore each other with no demands on either side. As well, these sequences give you specific permission to start telling your partner when something is not quite right, without her (or you) feeling awkward. Most importantly, they help you to get in touch with all your sensations, and start to expand your ability to experience them.

Begin by deciding who will be touched and who will be toucher.

Then get into a comfortable position; the touched could be lying on front or back with the toucher sitting beside them; the touched could be sitting back against the toucher's front; or you could be sitting opposite each other with open legs spread across each other.

Decide on any limits, or off-limits. We ask you, for the first sequence, not to touch each other's genitals. It also could be that one of you hates being touched on your ribs (it may tickle) or your feet (it may make you jump). You should agree that if the toucher does anything that doesn't feel good, the person being touched can say so, and the toucher will do something else, easily and silently.

STAGE 1

Begin touching. Do so for the pleasure you get out of it, the sight of your partner, the sound of her breathing or her voice, the sensations you get when you touch her; lean forward and smell and taste her skin and hair. Focus yourself on the sensations you have, and try to screen out all other sensations so that you are totally unaware of them. Be alert only to any sign from your partner that you are doing something that is not quite right for her. Keep touching, with all your senses involved, for about ten to fifteen minutes.

When it is time to swap over, relax as fully as you can before your partner touches you. Of course, you can tell her if there is anything you don't like, but otherwise simply concentrate on opening your senses as fully as possible. You may want to watch your partner – but you also may want to close your eyes and just concentrate on what you hear and feel. You may smell her as she leans forward. Remember that you do not have to give anything back; you can just enjoy exactly what you are experiencing.

If you start to feel aroused or to get an erection either as toucher or touched, for the moment let that go. When you have both taken you turn, then if you want to you can carry on to make love in the usual way. For the moment, ignore any arousal and don't act on it.

Perhaps you find yourself feeling negative as you do this exercise. Perhaps you feel that it is a waste of time, or you find your mind wandering; perhaps you feel nothing, or sudden anger against your partner. Begin by relaxing completely, breathing into the relaxation and focusing your mind on what you are feeling; often you are simply unused to accepting pleasure and simply need to give your body time to get used to that.

If the negative feelings persist, you may want to talk that through in case you have any unresolved issues that need sorting out with your partner. Perhaps there is a past memory of something that happened, with your partner or a previous lover, that is still blocking you from feeling pleasure. This is the chance to discuss it and lay ghosts to rest.

On the other hand, if you feel very relaxed, close and intimate perhaps suddenly relieved that you are feeling so much for each other, then tell your partner so and cuddle her in whatever way you want to.

Do this sequence several times together before passing on to Stage 2.

STAGE 2

The next stage is to focus your attention even more by beginning to communicate with your partner about what is happening, what you need and what you want. It involves touching each other again in exactly the same way as we have just described – but instead of only telling each other if something goes wrong, try also telling each other whenever something is particularly pleasurable. You might murmur, say a few words, groan all the codes you know to signify pleasure, and then a few more. Notice, how doing this increases the ability of the person touching to focus in on what is good and do that more. Notice, too, if you are being touched, how expressing your pleasure increases it.

Again, if any negative feelings come up,

discuss them with your partner. Make sure, if you do, that this doesn't take up the whole of the available time and lead to her missing her turn. Equally, if she feels uncomfortable and wants to talk things through with you, make sure you get your turn of being touched.

Repeat this sequence several times together over a few love-making sessions before passing on to Stage 3.

Stage 3

The final step is to begin to expand you repertoire. You have already focused on your feelings and on expanding your capacity for pleasure through relaxed touching. Now take it further.

Repeat the sequence, but this time use unexpected parts of your body to touch unexpected parts of hers: your unerect penis to lightly touch her back; her hair to brush the back of your neck, your fingernails to lightly scratch the inside of her thighs. Use unexpected things, though nothing hurtful: soft, sharp, warm, cold; feathers, strips of torn paper, even ice if you give your partner warning and use it gently; to touch, stroke, rub, tickle, scratch, press. Explore and experiment with the pressure and speed of your touch, the rhythm, and when to stop and start. Add extra lubrication and see what difference that makes.

Explore in particular what you could be doing with your mouth. Kissing on the lips you will know about, but what about kissing other parts of your partner's body – ears, wrists, backs of knees, soles of feet, insides of thighs, eyelids? And how do you kiss – softly, hard, breathing, with your tongue? Try licking or sucking instead of kissing. Use your teeth to nibble or bite gently. Experiment with dry kisses or wet ones – then blow over moistened skin for added sensation. How slow can you kiss, how rhythmically, and what happens when you stop kissing for the space of three heartbeats, and then start in again suddenly with no warning?

Of course, your whole body is an erogenous zone, but which are the most sensitive zones for your partner and for you? You can spend literally hours tracing all over each other to find unknown sensitive spots – and for her, certainly, the exercise can be endless, for at different times of the day, different times of the month, and in different moods, she will like things totally differently.

If you feel uncomfortable feeling so much pleasure, try relaxing as much as you can and letting it carry on. Do this sequence several times with your partner – and then begin each love-making session with at least several minutes of such undemanding touching. You will soon find the difference it makes to your sexuality.

SEXUAL TROUBLE-SHOOTING

Being sensuous with each other is not just a sexual enhancement tool, but also a vital first step in dissolving sexual blocks. So let us be clear about just how the explorations in this chapter will help you with specific problems.

- If your desire for each other has faded, then the non-demand methods we suggest here will help you both learn what you and your partner really need, without any pressure to perform.

- If you are feeling sexual boredom, the sequences will allow you to start being clear with each other about what you want and don't want, a key issue when boredom occurs.

- They will also help overcome in you or your partner any unwillingness to simply let go and feel pleasure.

SUPERVIRILITY

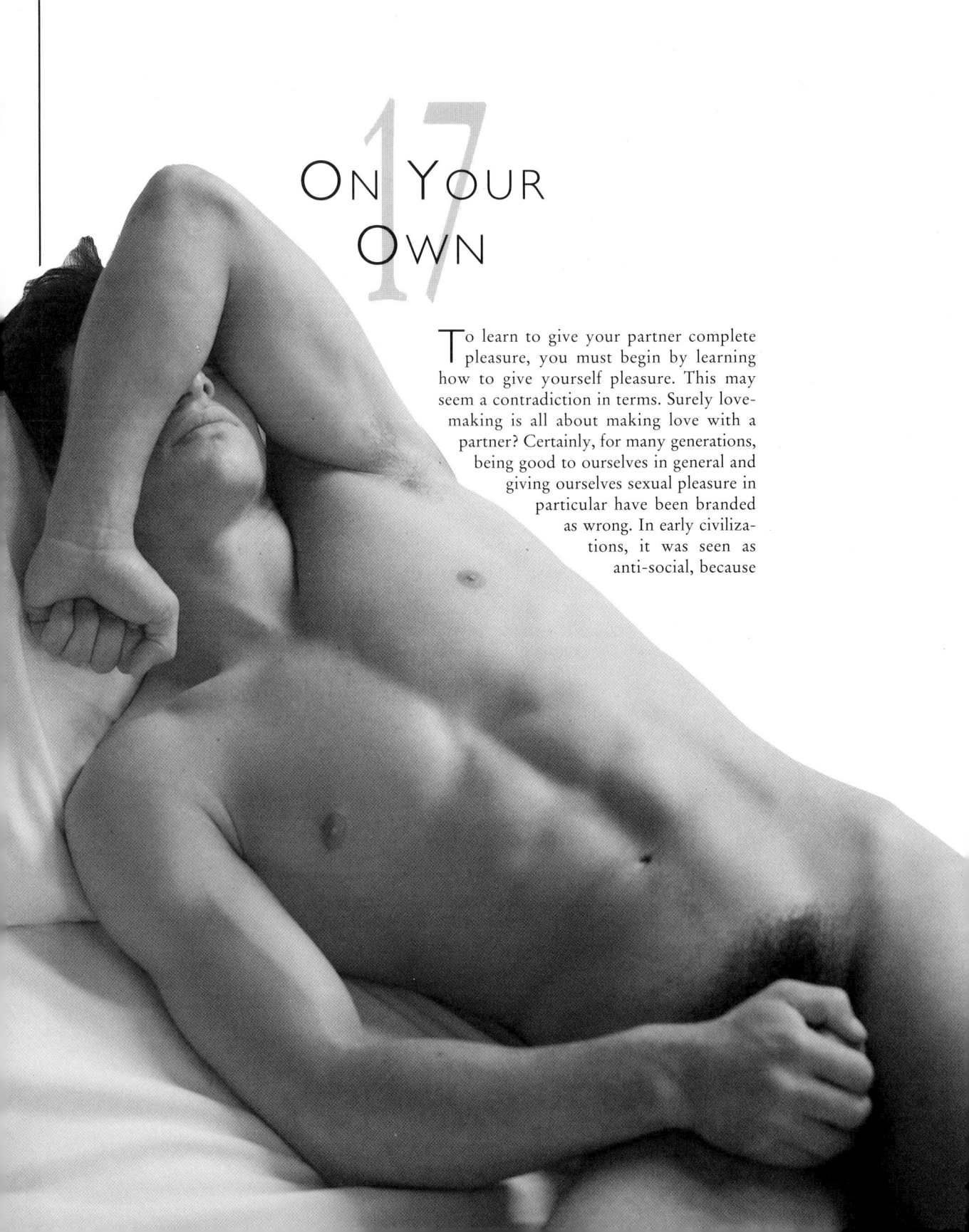

17 ON YOUR OWN

To learn to give your partner complete pleasure, you must begin by learning how to give yourself pleasure. This may seem a contradiction in terms. Surely lovemaking is all about making love with a partner? Certainly, for many generations, being good to ourselves in general and giving ourselves sexual pleasure in particular have been branded as wrong. In early civilizations, it was seen as anti-social, because it 'spilled the seed'. In Victorian times, it was seen as immoral and against God. And even very recently, when psychologists began to explore sexuality, masturbation was regarded as immature, essentially self-focused and precluding love for another person.

Thankfully now all these myths have – on the surface at any rate – been laid to rest. They still lurk in our minds, though, for we may well as boys have been told off for touching ourselves, or been caught embarrassed with our hand under the sheet and a copy of *Playboy* on the pillow.

But self-pleasuring is essential in a number of ways. It teaches you how your body and your sexuality work, allows you to rehearse for love-making with your partner, lets you find out what sensations most turn you on. Through allowing you the time and opportunity to experiment, it allows you to begin to explore just how you can increase your possible arousal. With a partner, often you feel you have not the freedom to experiment; with a partner, the pressure is on to move love-making to its conclusion, or to put your attention on her rather than on yourself. So although all sex is about self-discovery, sometimes you can initially discover more alone than you can together.

Finally, if you have a sexual block, masturbation is often the place to start. By taking time alone to recreate the situation where blocks may arise, you can explore them, familiarize yourself with them and so begin to overcome them.

So give yourself permission to please yourself.

STARTING OFF

Set aside time regularly to spend alone masturbating. Make this as often as you want to, perhaps once a day, perhaps once a week. Your hormone levels are highest first thing in the morning, but you may not have time; bear in mind, too, that if you masturbate to orgasm, you may have longer to wait before you can get it up with your partner. If you can be open with your partner about what you are doing, then so much the better – if not, make sure that you choose to be somewhere where there is no fear of interruption by anyone, and somewhere you will be at ease. This may not be your bedroom, but unlike partner sex, which is often lusciously risky taken in the kitchen or the countryside, the sort of exploratory masturbation we are recommending may need real privacy.

Make yourself comfortable – try to contradict the messages you may have received from childhood which said that masturbation had to be done in a rushed manner in the most uncomfortable place possible! Just as you would for love-making, find a comfortable rug, sofa or bed, make sure you have support for your back if that is important for you, and at least to begin with, have at hand any particular objects that you may need. Many men do like to rub up against something when they masturbate. Give yourself dim lighting, music, cushions, erotica to start you off, some incense to make the room smell nice. Lubrication is often useful too, and although you can use your own saliva, baby oil is a nice alternative. Beware of using oils that are perfumed as we ourselves know to our cost that on delicate parts of one's anatomy they can sting like crazy! A box of paper hankies may also be necessary for afterwards.

Begin by exploring your own body, perhaps in front of the mirror, perhaps by touch alone and with your eyes shut. Don't just leap for the genitals, however much you feel that that is where the urgency is. Instead, experiment with different kinds of touches on different parts of your body; the sensitive skin of your ears, the inside of your elbows, even the soles of your feet. How does each part of your body feel to you, and how does your touch affect it? Rehearse different kinds of touches, becoming aware of how they affect you and therefore how they may affect your partner when you touch her. Move on after a while to your genitals; touch your penis, your testicles, the inside of your thighs, and back to your anus. Take time to contrast what effect different touches have on you. Which areas of your genitals are most sensitive, which seem not to respond?

You may well have begun to get aroused. Notice what that feels like, and where you feel it in your body. Perhaps without your noticing it, your penis has begun to erect. But don't aim for that. The secret at present is to concentrate on the sensations beginning to flood your senses.

Moving On

Stage 1

Move slowly on to direct arousal. You may want to begin with your usual method of masturbation, taking up the position which is best for you, on your back or stomach, perhaps sitting up or on your side; ease gradually into the movement which you usually need, easing the foreskin back and forth if that is good for you.

As you move, begin to become aware of what works best. Make a mental note of exactly what you need in order to begin to be aroused, in terms of position, speed, pressure, rhythm, movement – as well as in terms of where you are and how you feel emotionally. If you notice something isn't working and is holding you back, don't dwell on that; it is a sign to change what you are doing to something else, so immediately move on and try something different.

What if, at this stage, you get no response at all? Check out that your mental state is secure – if you know that your three-year-old child is going to come bursting in at any moment, or you are expecting a phone call from your boss, it would be very surprising if an erection came easily! Equally, check out if there is anything that is putting you off: the state of the room, the worry about erection, the game on the television. If all seems fine, first relax as completely as you can, then try upping the ante: add in some further lubrication, try changing your grip, or concentrate for a while on the most luscious fantasy you can. But don't make it a life or death thing – your body may simply not be in the mood. Try again tomorrow, and each day until you do get some response and can then try experimenting more fully with what suits.

STAGE 2

The next stage is to learn to play with your erection, to find out your pleasure limits and then go beyond them, to take full control over your body and its capacity for arousal.

Begin by arousing yourself to the point of erection, then as soon as you feel any stiffening, stop. Stop whatever you are doing, thinking, feeling or imagining, and let your erection die. There may be a sense of panic as you do this; it is an extremely unusual thing, to deliberately choose to watch your erection fade. If you do feel any resistance to doing it, use the deep-breathing techniques that we suggest in Chapter 15 to fully relax yourself and your body.

Once your erection has faded, begin again to stimulate yourself. Use all the things that you know work. And once again, as you reach erection (which may be a matter of a few seconds or may take an hour) then stop and let it subside.

Why do we suggest this? Allowing your erection to fade away does several things, on a physical and on a mental level. Firstly, the usual practice of masturbating to orgasm furiously and in a task-oriented manner means that, in fact, although pleasure is high at the time, there is no learning involved. More often than not, you simply don't get to find out whether what you did works well, better or best – or whether doing something slightly differently could be giving you a different sensation. You don't get to expand your repertoire of stimulation, of ways to get to erection, of pleasure, because once you start to get aroused you are just concerned about getting there.

Secondly, because there is a tendency to pounce on an erection and take it to orgasm as soon as it appears, all too often it feels transitory. It seems in some way to come from heaven, with no control over what is happening. By allowing it to fail and then bringing it back again, you can discover what you need to do to make happen again, and you can also begin to reassure yourself that you can do it again, and again. You insure your psyche against the mental panic that has been mentioned throughout this book as the underlying cause of much sexual angst.

Bring yourself to erection and then let it die away three times. Then, if you want to, bring yourself off. Repeat this sequence from start to finish for several days before going on to the next step.

STAGE 3

Once you are happy that you have control over your erection, and once you have fully mastered the idea of experimenting with new ways of stimulating yourself, then you can go on to the next stage.

As before, gain an erection. Then, instead of letting it die, carry on. Continue using all the ways that you now know to arouse yourself until you reach the plateau phase – the point just before orgasm when you are not quite at the point of no return. Be aware of just when this is – you may well need a few practices before you can catch yourself before reaching this point, rather than going over it and into orgasm.

Conversely, if you find difficulty reaching this point, particularly if you feel that you may never come, then be sure you are paying attention to what you need in the way we suggested before. Are you in the right position, using the right movement, concentrating on the right fantasy? Is everything right for you? You may want to add in extra stimulation, too, with firmer strokes, more pressure or added lubrication.

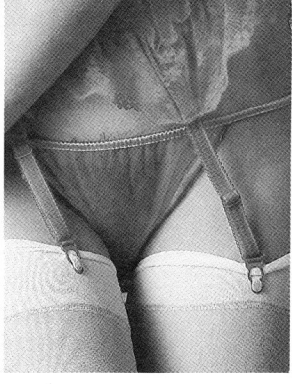

But don't push things; if you sometimes find it difficult to get aroused, then reaching this stage may take you several times of trying. Practice deep relaxation so that you do not enter an anxiety spiral.

When you do reach the plateau phase, just at the moment when you sense that you are about to come, again stop what you are doing and let your erection die away completely.

Once more, you may feel strange doing this – don't worry if you can't achieve it the first time you try. All your senses may scream to you to go on. But as soon as you can, stop. Take your hands away, leave your erection alone. Use deep breathing to fully relax. Keep thinking that soon you will be arousing yourself again. Don't use the traditional counting techniques to switch yourself off; they tend to distract you from sensation. Deep relaxation works far better, keeping you in touch with what is happening and what your body is doing all the time.

When your erection is completely down, start again. Experiment with how you can develop different sensations in your penis or in other parts of your body. Learn to trust that you can bring yourself off as slowly as you like, and that you have a choice over whether to come or not. When you have successfully been able to bring yourself backwards and forwards from the plateau phase three times, use increased stimulation to bring yourself off – noticing as you do so the difference in sensation you feel from when you simply go for it the first time. (If you have difficulty going over threshold to orgasm, then it is fine not to orgasm.)

Repeat this sequence several times, over a period of several days, before going further.

STAGE 4

Finally, you should have learned a great deal about what pleases you. You should also feel far more comfortable about the non-urgency of having an erection. You will almost certainly, by this time, be starting to differentiate different sensations with different types of masturbation. You will also by this time be starting to experience deeper and deeper orgasms when they happen.

The next stage is to begin to explore how far you can extend your ability to accept pleasure before you come. There is no need, once you are confident, to take yourself all the way back to non-erection once you reach the point of no return; simply stop or slow down for a little while, until you feel you are well back from the brink, and then start in again. However much stimulation it has taken you to get there, hovering in the plateau phase can be extended and enhanced, as you play with pleasure, increasing and decreasing it, teasing yourself towards and away from the edge.

And add in extra elements, as you feel able to accept them without crossing the brink. Use erotica, fantasy – and these two extra suggestions.

- **Use a vibrator.** There are a variety, some to strap on the back of the hand, others shaped like phalluses, with interchangeable heads. Buy them at sex shops or by mail order; large retail chemists often do them disguised tactfully as 'massagers'. If yours has been bought by your partner for her use, you may have to go with what she has chosen; but, if not, you may find that some shapes are better for you than others! Vibrators vary in the electrical frequency they use, though the most effective seem to be those at about 80Hz, mains operated. As with cock rings that use current, don't worry about electricity near private parts, as the current is too low to be harmful. You can often get the best results by putting the head of the vibrator against the underside of the head of your penis, where it is most sensitive; experiment to find exactly where is right for you. Try gentle strokes, different rhythms, or simply press the vibrator firmly into the penis.

- **Use sensation enhancement.** This is a technique taken from the new psychological approach of Neuro-Linguistic Programming (NLP). First concentrate on each sense in turn – sight, sound, smell, taste, touch. As you concentrate, imagine having a 'graphic equalizer' on each sense, so that you can turn sensation up and up, but can stop if you start to feel panicky because things are going too fast for you. Edge the control up just a little each time. Then close your eyes and concentrate on your arousal, until it blocks out all other senses – shut out any extraneous sounds, for example, or any words you are saying to yourself. Again imagine there is a graphic equalizer on your arousal, and you are turning it up and up until you can stand no more.

End every session with an orgasm; and notice how, when you finally tip over the edge, the sensation will be increasingly stronger.

SEXUAL TROUBLE-SHOOTING

The prime aim of the sexual explorations in this chapter is to develop your capacity for pleasure. But you will also find that they gradually whittle away at any sexual blocks.

- If your desire has faded, or boredom has set in, then the step-by-step methods we suggest here will help you get back in touch with what you really need in sex; by taking the pressure off having to perform for your partner, they will also help you re-ignite your sexual longing.

- By encouraging you to learn about your own erection, and by allowing you practice in regaining that erection, they will allow you to regain trust in your own body functions and overcome any anxiety about your performance.

- By building the pleasure in the plateau stage, they begin to take the emphasis off the importance of coming.

- And equally, by letting you know that you can bring yourself back to this stage, they begin to build the confidence that will allow you to tip over the edge into orgasm when you choose to.

- If you do have difficulty in any of these areas, then letting go of your erection may stir panic in you. Don't let it. Relax deeply, and take your time. It may take months to really get to know your body and its capacity for pleasure – for this is a generative rather than a remedial programme. You are not just learning to solve your problems; you are learning a whole new way of sexuality.

GETTING IT UP

If you have practised the arousal techniques of pushing yourself forward and holding yourself back, you will know exactly what you need in order to gain an erection.

But transferring these skills to the context of your partnership may still create blocks. For, mentally and emotionally, making love to yourself is a very different thing from making love to your partner – and many a man who cannot get an erection in the context of partnership sex is nevertheless able to have one easily on his own.

The first issue is that making love with a partner brings in all kinds of anxieties. But secondly, many men who wouldn't dream of trying to get an erection during masturbation by just sitting and hoping will expect spontaneous magic to happen if they are with their partner; their inner belief is that getting help with an erection if their partner is in the room is cheating – that if they really loved her, it would happen all by itself.

This is rubbish; it is particularly rubbish as time passes. For, with age, erections do start to need help. Physically, they are totally possible – but they don't leap up as they used to without some care and attention. And, if you still hang on to the belief that erections in love-making just happen, that you have no choice when they arrive, that you have to grin and bear it if they depart, that you cannot choose how long they last, and that you and your partner have no ability to create or enhance them, then you have a lot to learn.

You need to give your erection care and attention, and you need to learn to let your partner do the same. Real love-making involves both of you, and using all your resources to enhance erection is just as much a co-operative venture as using both your bodies to create an orgasm! We would go further. Allowing your partner to help you right from the start, in getting you up 'from cold' so to speak, is not only more involving for her and more relaxing for you; it also creates a more equal sexual relationship, where you and she together are taking responsibility for what is happening.

SHOWING HER HOW

First, however, a warning. The explorations in this book should remove most of the distress and worry about not being able to get it up. However, at any time, either with or without your partner, you may still have the occasional episode of erectile difficulty – through tiredness, strain or a sudden, inexplicable loss of confidence. Simply stop, relax, breathe deeply and cuddle for a while – and turn to some other way of getting sensual pleasure. The vital thing is to take the emphasis off performance; after that, your body will look after itself.

And, of course, if you need to, go back to the very start of the explorations in this section (Chapter 15) and work through them slowly, taking your time, until you get your confidence back.

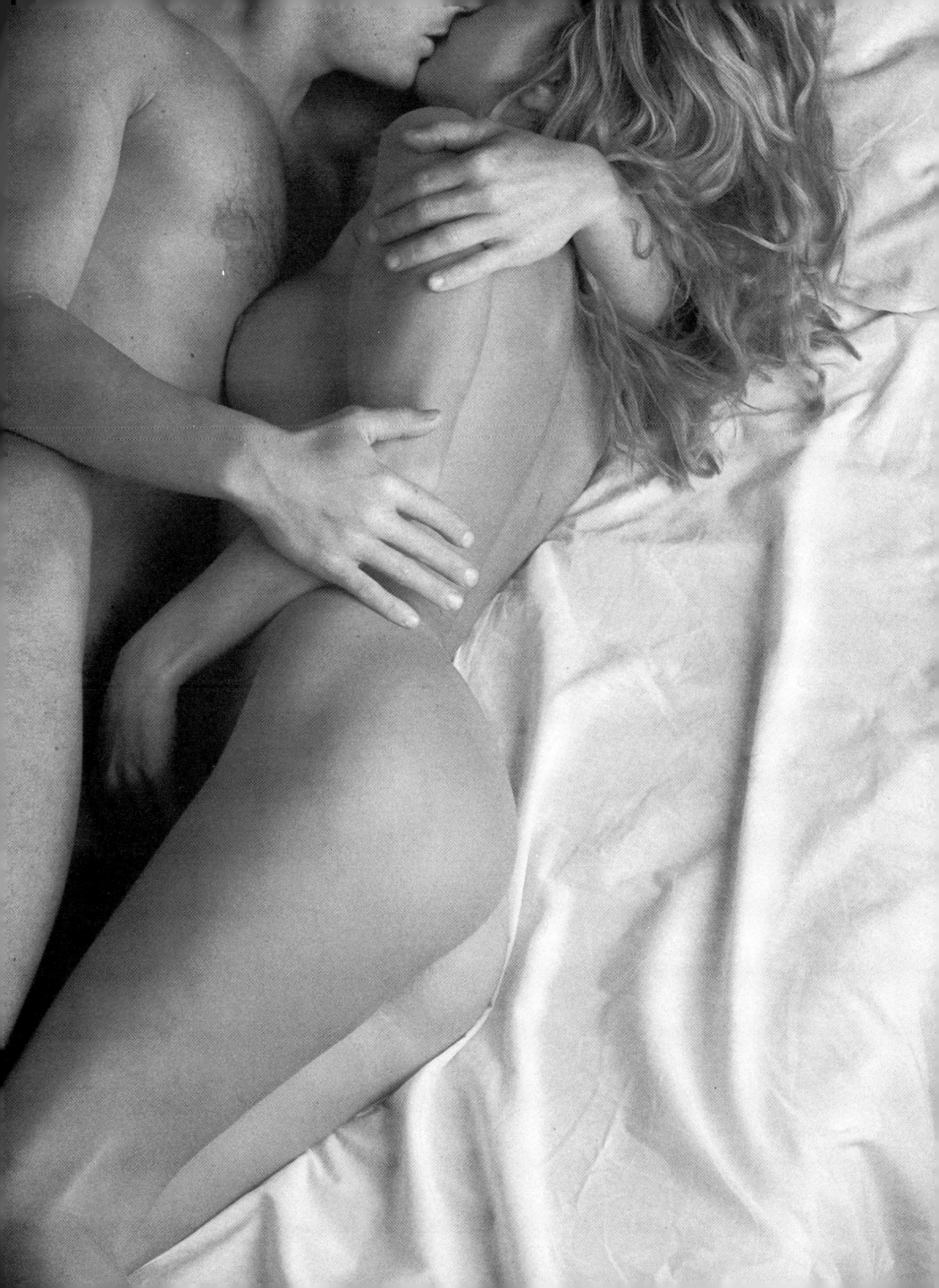

Next, you are going to show your partner just what you learned while you were pleasuring yourself. Some people, women as well as men, find it embarrassing to show their partner their masturbation style; if you feel like this, do relax – and set the scene. Decide first which position you want to be in. You may choose to lie flat on your back, be sitting up and supported by cushions, or half and half. Pick up on the positions you know from masturbation work best for you, and adapt them to suit. Don't hesitate to parallel your masturbation experience in love-making. The key at this stage is to take what you already know works and keep doing it.

At this stage, there is a temptation. Because you may be a little embarrassed, you may revert to pre-Supervirility habits. You may do it all quickly and surreptitiously, get it over and done with, and turn to your partner with a smile of triumph. This is not the way. In order to really know how to make love to you, she needs to learn your speeds and rhythms. She needs to know how you hold yourself back and then push yourself on again, how far-reaching your pleasure threshold is, just how much you can take.

So take a long time and make it lascivious. Let your partner involve herself in whatever way she likes to begin with, simply watching, kissing you, talking dirty. You are going to be doing this a lot, so she doesn't need to watch everything you do all at the same time. Don't fall into the trap of imagining this is a one-off learning experience. This should be an integral part of your love-making from now on. So use it for pleasure from the start.

Be aware, by the way, that if you have any sexual blocks that are underpinned by a need for control, or by feeling that sex is a bit dirty or messy, the step of masturbating in front of your partner may be a crucial one for you. Take it slowly. Begin by sitting close to your partner, maybe back to back, so that you can feel her comfortably supporting you, but you know she can't see you. Masturbate as usual, even if this means rubbing up against some object; it is more important to get aroused than to make contact with your partner at this point.

Practise this a number of times until you are comfortable with it. Gradually, move to a different position so that you are holding your partner against you as you masturbate – and then, each time you masturbate, move a little closer so that she is eventually watching you. If you need reassurance while you are masturbating, be aware of her love, and how she gets turned on by your arousal. Again, practise as often as you need to until ejaculating in front of your partner is easy, comfortable and arousing.

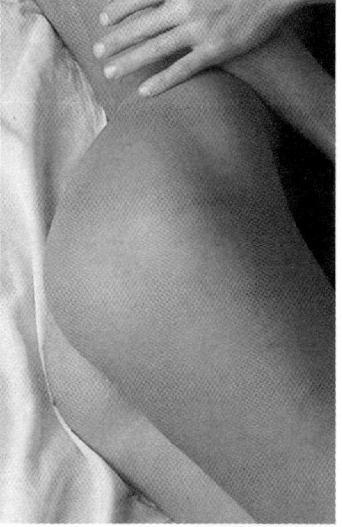

HER TURN

There will come a time, fairly soon, when with your partner beside you, you can arouse yourself, hold yourself back, keep yourself going and then take your orgasm. Then is the time when she can start to get more involved. At first, she can kiss, lick, move against you. You may want to allow yourself to do simply this for a while, as she slowly starts to take over the movements of masturbation herself.

If your partner has never brought you off before, then what she does will be largely learned from what you have done. At first, she should follow carefully what you have shown her, learning exactly and precisely what works for you, so that she can replicate it as and when needed.

Then, she can begin to experiment. If, as is likely with a long-term partner, she is used to bringing you off, then encourage her at this stage to try out her own inspirations. It could be that none of her experiments are suitable for you – and just as you told her what wasn't good when you were touching each other's bodies, so you have to be very precise about what doesn't work when she is bringing you off. Don't jump in immediately with an 'Oh, that's no good' but as soon as you are sure that what she is doing is getting you less rather than more aroused, then say so lovingly. Equally, do be prepared to accept her experiments; there will be things that are a total failure when you do them to yourself that send you sky high when she does them. Sexual fulfilment is not about following a tried and tested route.

What are your partner's options? We are tempted to leave you simply to let her experiment, as this will create the possibility of some moves that we have never even thought of. However, here are some clues.

STAGE 1

Let her start with her hand, perhaps, holding your penis in the way you like it held, stroking it between tip and root. Let her manipulate it like a roll of plastic, or run well-lubricated fingers around the head of the penis. Let her use both hands, just two fingers, the palm of her hand on the tip. Let her, if you are uncircumcised, ease the foreskin back and forth over the glans. Let her vary speed, pressure, rhythm and all those elements that you have identified are crucial to your pleasure. Let her, at the same time, not forget your testicles – or the rest of your body, mouth, nipples and other sensitive spots.

Then, she may want to use her mouth. Keeping her teeth out of the way, she may want to plunge your penis into her mouth, lick it as if it were an ice cream, slide her tongue round the tip, or vigorously stimulate the frenulum. She may want to suck, allowing your penis to slide easily into her mouth, but then firmly holding it between her lips as it emerges. She may want to suck your testicles, taking them gently into her mouth one at a time.

Whether you react to all this by coming immediately or merely by stiffening slightly will all depend not only on your partner and what she is doing, but also on whether you are used to her touch and to her giving you oral sex. If you know you have blocks about being comfortable with your partner being involved, take it slowly. A first time can be mind-blowing, or merely feel strange. A thousandth time may be comfortable or suddenly ecstatic.

STAGE 2

But, however you react, once your partner has gained an even partial erection for you, you will want to slow the whole thing down and start allowing yourself to enjoy more pleasure. Again, the secret is to begin by getting her to use her hands and mouth to bring you erect from cold, and as soon as she has done this, to allow yourself to diminish. (Your partner will need to know just why, as stopping suddenly can feel strange even if you are not on the receiving end!)

As your erection diminishes, just talk or cuddle; don't turn your attention away from each other, but keep non-arousing contact. As soon as you are down, you can start again. As previously, you need to let your erection die several times in order to build your confidence in your erection and to give your partner time to practise.

STAGE 3

Once you are confident, you can continue on to the next stage as you did when you were masturbating, building up to the plateau phase and then allowing your erection to die. Again, if you feel yourself going over the edge, you must signal to your partner, who should stop and back away. In time, she herself will be able to tell when you are getting ready to come, and back off herself.

If you find that you are coming without warning, then an extra weapon in her armoury is this technique, used for 1400 years in China to avoid ejaculation. She places her fingers one each side of your frenulum, and squeezes for five to ten seconds. This usually pulls you back from coming and then she can ease away and give you a chance to climb down from the plateau phase.

Again, you should become proficient in being able to come back down from the point of no return before moving on to the next stage.

STAGE 4

With each experience of being able to hold yourself in the plateau phase, you will be able to tolerate more and more pleasure. There is no need to let your erection die completely now; once you are at the point of no return, simply stop or slow down until you come slightly away from that point, and then begin again.

SEXUAL TROUBLE-SHOOTING

As before, all these explorations will also help you if you have a particular sexual block. Specifically:

- Your desire will be enhanced by flooding your senses with stimulation, particularly when you involve your partner and so have a whole new set of stimuli affecting you.

- Any mental tendency you have to lose your erection will be helped by you and your partner learning together that you can create and maintain it when you want to; of course, any time that you feel uncertain about your erection, go back to what we suggest in this chapter and the previous ones and use it enthusiastically!

- If by any chance you do have premature ejaculation, you will get more control; in particular, the squeeze technique that your partner learns will come in useful, having the added advantage that through it she can let you know when she needs you to last longer.

- If delayed ejaculation is your problem, then the act of holding back from ejaculation will help you learn that you are in charge of it.

- Particularly, working with your partner to simply receive pleasure is a total contradiction of all the performance issues that we have looked at throughout the book. For Supervirility, you need to learn that, sometimes, it is **OK** to lie back and let your partner pleasure you; and that in doing so, in the long run you provide a more fulfilling sex life for both of you.

Getting It Up

Now, begin to add in further stimulation. Make sure your partner is touching you on other parts of your body that get you further turned on. Begin more slowly, using erotica or any of the pre-erection techniques we mentioned to prolong the agony! Help yourself by touching yourself or her in various ways. Add extra lubrication. Let her use a vibrator in whichever way she wants. And don't forget to use your mind to enhance your sexuality. Use sensory enhancement. Contact your most erotic fantasies, or get her to tell you hers.

As always, each time you make love, you should practise these steps, ending always if you want to in orgasms for one or both of you. But again, as always, don't panic if orgasm doesn't come.

Your potential for being able to depend on it will increase in direct proportion to the amount you carry out these explorations.

A final word. If you know you are using these techniques to trouble-shoot rather than simply to enhance your sexuality, there is at this stage one very important limitation. You should be holding back from intercourse – that is, until you are easily and pleasurably carrying out all the suggestions in this chapter, and pushing your pleasure barriers to the limit. This may seem odd, but holding back from intercourse is an essential part of sexual trouble-shooting. You need to feel you are not under pressure to perform. So stay away from full intercourse until you have worked through all these explorations.

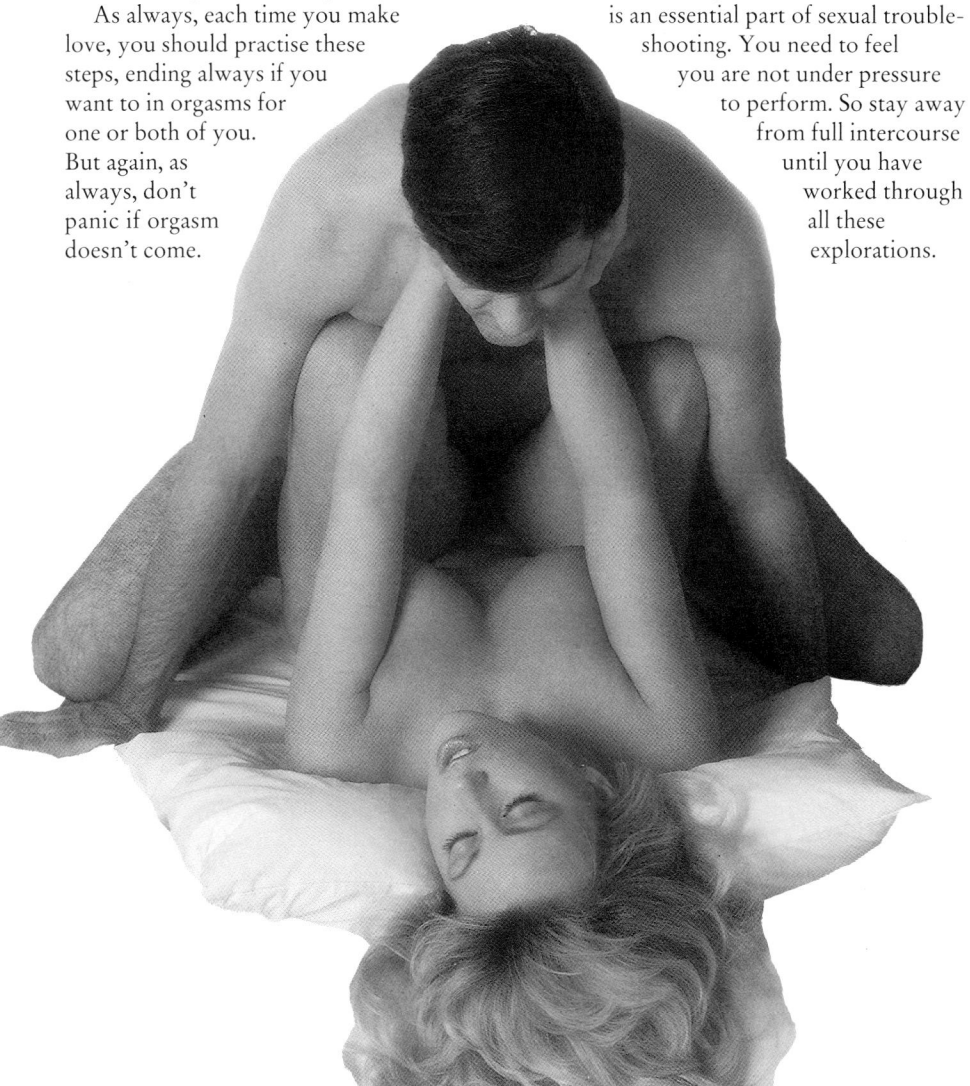

Pleasure without Penetration

There is a world of enjoyment that lies between arousal and orgasm that never involves intercourse. Whether or not you have an erection that will penetrate, whether or not your partner likes to have your penis inside her, there are a variety of ways to further arouse you both.

Her Pleasure

The first step is to find out what your partner needs, how she can be given the most possible pleasure. Perhaps she has been following you in your explorations into the senses, seeing you holding yourself back and then pushing yourself on. We hope – though this is not the book that specifically teaches women Supervirility skills – that she has adapted some of these techniques for herself. (If your partner is as yet unable to come at all, then see Chapter 14.) Maybe she has learned to prolong her pleasure in orgasm, has learned to masturbate herself quickly and easily to a climax.

So the first step is to find out from her how she does this. Just as she needed to learn anew what you liked, so you now need to learn all over again just what pleases her.

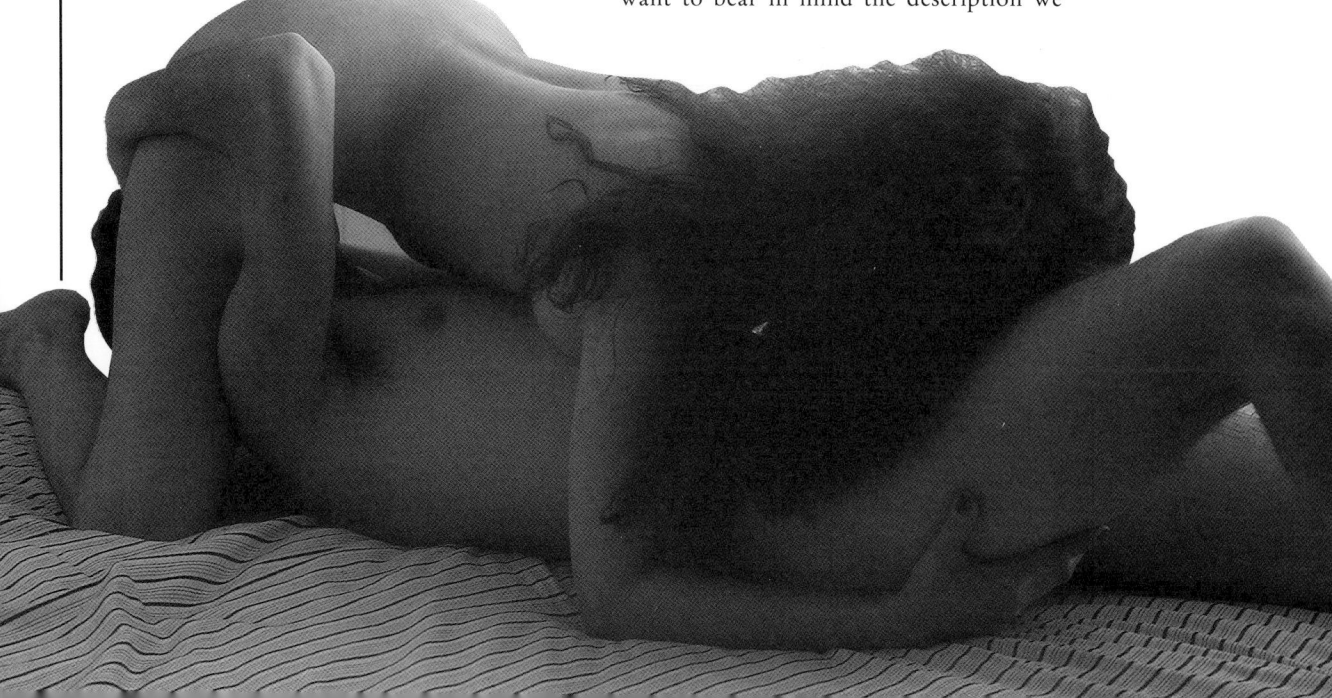

If she is willing, get her to teach you in the same way as you taught her – by showing you. First of all, once you are both relaxed and feeling sensuous in the way we describe in Chapter 15, take the opportunity to explore her genitals gently and lovingly, looking, feeling, tasting and smelling, getting her to give you a running commentary on what feels nice. You may want to bear in mind the description we give of her genitals in Chapter 14, making sure you know which part is which. She may want to join you in this exploration, with a mirror if that helps her to see what she is touching.

Then support her to lie or sit in the right position, to touch herself in the best way, to add in extra stimulation as she needs it. Watch what she does, and learn from it. Check her position, her movements, her speed and her rhythm. Take particular note of where she likes anything that may be the direct opposite of what you like, an irregular rhythm where you want insistent thrusting, a slow pace where you prefer it fast. Notice whether she touches only her clitoris, or whether she needs to insert her fingers into her vagina, whether she rubs herself against anything or needs to touch her breasts.

But, as with you, don't let things stop there. She may have another position, another set of movements, another way or ways of coming that she uses at other times, when the sensations in her vagina are different, or when her level of arousal is higher or lower. So encourage her to masturbate with you not once but several times; more than that, make it a regular and integral part of your love-making.

You need not be just an observer; you can make your watching an erotic experience by whispering fantasies to her. You can kiss her while she moves. You can stroke her breasts, her thighs and her face as she comes, and if, like you, she is working on holding herself back, bringing herself on, extending her ability to stay in the plateau phase, you can hold on to her as she stops herself, and then stay with her as she carries on. One couple we know, who are frighteningly 'equal' out of bed, include in their love-making rituals one where she brings herself off – but he dictates when she stops and starts, judging from her moans just when she is on the edge, and then making her wait and wait until she pleads with him for permission to carry on.

JOINING IN

When you are both at ease with her masturbating herself, and when you both know that learning about her masturbation skills is an essential part of your love-making, you can move on to joining in. You can start to touch her, and tongue her.

As you do so, leave behind all your preconceptions. Forget what you think works for her; instead, concentrate on replicating what she did to herself. With your finger, follow hers (place your hand over hers to learn) with the exact position and movement she uses. When you use your tongue, repeat her finger movements, rhythm, and speed as you flick, probe or vibrate. If she likes fingers penetrating her vagina, do that. How much lubrication does she need – and should that be her own saliva, or extra oil? Ease her into the position she best likes, and add to all that any extra touches – kisses, stroking, words, that you know she responds to.

For the moment, don't use your initiative; concentrate on really learning what she wants. So many people, when bringing their partners off, regard it as something that must be continued regardless. If you stop, then that is a failure of skill or nerve; far better to carry on as if you knew what you were doing. Others believe that, having been with the same partner for years, asking or checking is a failure of knowledge or love. These attitudes are not Supervirility. Supervirility is slowly and constantly updating your knowledge of each other. And remember that, once you have mastered one of her ways of masturbating herself, then you may well want to learn the other ways, too – until you know them all and can use them as and when necessary, switching from one to another as her mood and her physiology change.

Once you have mastered her technique, and know that you can bring her to orgasm regularly, then you can start to experiment.

She will know by this time that her orgasm is assured, so she will be able to relax and allow you to vary what you do. Change position, change the movement, and each time see what happens. Alter the speed, pressure and rhythm, not just once, but many times. Explore her vagina, her clitoris; add in extra hand or tongue stimulation on her thighs, breasts, mouth.

If your partner is willing, you can use Supervirility techniques to expand her pleasure potential, too. Once you feel that she is aroused, stop for just a moment and then carry on. Once you have the sense that she is in the plateau phase, let things die for just a moment, and then increase the pleasure – more movement, more pressure, more sensation. Get her to the point where only just one more stroke would take her over the edge; let her slide down again to a point below that; then work her up again, slowly.

Remember that at this stage while pleasure for you often means more – more pressure, more speed, more strength – for some women pleasure means less: a touch so light she can hardly feel it, a rhythm so irregular that she has no idea where the next stroke is coming from. After you have mastered all this, of course, you can add in as much stimulation as she can stand – and this does not have to be from you. Like you, she can fantasize in her mind as you bring her off; like you, she can use sensory enhancement techniques to raise her arousal level. And you can add to the possibilities.

Use the shower attachment very gently on her clitoris. Try all the non-erection techniques we used in Chapter 16, such as stroking her with feathers, or gently scratching with short nails. Use a vibrator on her, stimulating her clitoris first and, if it is a penis-shaped vibrator, then entering her if she wants that. Dildos, an ancient sex toy used in Eastern harems, are another option; use them in her anus or her vagina (but not one after the other, as infection can occur that way). They are especially useful if, for any reason, she wants penetration but you are unable or unwilling to supply it this time round. Use any of these extra forms of stimulation as she moves in and out of the plateau phase, and then use them all together to push her over the edge.

YOUR PLEASURE TOGETHER

By now, having each learned what it takes to bring the other to the plateau phase and hold them there, you can move on to mutual love-making, combining the two.

There is more than some discussion about whether it is really possible to masturbate each other mutually all the way to orgasm. Certainly if one of you is deeply into the plateau phase, they have very little attention for careful hand or tongue work. That said, particularly in the early stages, mutual masturbation can be totally ecstatic, containing all the elements of mutuality that make penetration so attractive, whilst at the same time having all the clitoral stimulation that for her may be a peak experience of sex.

Begin by finding a position that suits you. For hand jobs, side by side on your backs is probably as good a position as any, with arms overlapping. Try top-to-toe, or soixante-neuf, with each of you lying on your side with each other's knee forming a pillow for the other's head. This position is usually used for mouth jobs, but works just as well if you are using your hands. The alternative is for one of you to lie on their back, with the other kneeling over them, genitals to mouth; the classic is with her on top, but depending on your relative sizes, you on top can work just as well.

Or, she can lie on her back on the bed with you in her mouth, while your hands reach down and over her. An alternative that misses true mutuality, though it may provide the element of self-control that is needed, is that she offers you her mouth in such a position that you can move to your rhythm inside her. Meanwhile, she alone, or she guiding your hand, stimulates her clitoris.

Once you have moved into these positions, allow yourselves a little time to adjust. You will need to accustom yourselves to what each of you need. It could be that the required speed and rhythm are the same, and that you can move together and in unison; here your non-verbal 'codes' will really come into their own. More likely, you will need to move to different rhythms, for what you want in terms of speed or pressure may not be what she wants and, for each of you, keeping up the stimulation that the other wants may be difficult if you are trying to focus on your own arousal. Because of this, one of you may need to 'lie back and enjoy yourself', giving only token stimulation until they reach orgasm; after a while, you can reverse roles.

However, this can work to your advantage, given the Supervirility principles. You could, perhaps, get her to stimulate you from non-erection to erection this way, then lie back and let your erection die while you arouse her with your tongue. Several turns of this may bring you both to the point where you can be quickly and easily aroused to the plateau phase, after which you can again play with taking turns, one stimulating while the other lies completely still, and receives, then vice versa.

In the end, although simultaneous orgasm is rarely achievable this way, perhaps one of you could tongue the other to climax while at the same time bringing themselves off with their hand. As with every sequence we suggest in this entire final section of the book, mutual masturbation needs some sessions spent on it. Experiment with bringing each other from non-arousal to full arousal, then letting it all die away and beginning again.

Experiment with bringing each other to the edge of orgasm, then letting it die away either just a little; gradually extend your skill and your ability to handle pleasure using these techniques. As always, if possible, end each session with an orgasm for you, and at least one for her.

SEXUAL TROUBLE-SHOOTING

It may seem as if giving your partner pleasure and mutual masturbation have little to do with sexual blocks. In fact, both are stages not only in enhancing your sexuality, but also in giving you control and confidence in trouble-shooting.

- Fading desire on either of your sides may well be underpinned by your partner's lack of pleasure in lovemaking; being able to rely on giving each other hand or mouth orgasms can dramatically revitalize sexuality for you both and in particular may give her the pleasure she needs.

- The same is true if you have been suffering boredom. The added element of mutuality in simultaneous or consecutive masturbation can bring back not only desire but interest.

- The explorations we offer here continue to give you confidence about erection simply by making you more at ease with losing and gaining it in increasingly intimate situations.

- Learning to hold back even with the greatly enhanced stimulation of oral sex will help any hint of premature ejaculation.

- And the incredibly erotic sensations of mutual masturbation will give you enhanced love-making that takes the worry away from any likelihood that you will not come.

Pleasure with Penetration

Supervirility certainly doesn't focus on intercourse – but it does value it.

The biological reasons for intercourse (as a way to make babies) may be irrelevant to you; equally, the sexual justification for intercourse (as a way to orgasm) may be irrelevant to your partner. But it is still a nice thing to do. And if you can learn not only to take increasing pleasure from penetration and intercourse yourself and give increasing pleasure to your partner, its intimacy value, as you meet in the closest way imaginable, can be unparalleled.

Preparing for Penetration

As you move towards penetration, certain questions arise. Should you wait until your partner is well lubricated with vaginal fluid? For her, it is almost certainly better to wait until she is very aroused and therefore probably wet. For you, it could be that the drier she is, the more stimulation you get, and if you are unsure in any way of your erection, then this friction may be invaluable.

Equally, should you penetrate erect or non-erect? The traditional way is to only go for penetration when your erection is hard – but, in fact, you can not only use intercourse as a means to get an erection, you can also harden up an ambivalent erection by going for penetration early. Our suggestion is that, for the purposes of developing your Supervirility, you learn how to penetrate limp. You then have the choice. You can go for penetration as soon as you or your partner wants to, and build up arousal from there.

One good way to start is with your partner on top; she can squat or kneel over your penis, balancing herself with one hand to leave the other free for insertion. This position gives her the control to move in a way that is best for her and allows you to lie back and enjoy it if you want to. Either of you could perhaps use fingers at the base of your penis to act as a kind of tourniquet, so you can stiffen it slightly to insert into her vagina.

An alternative is what is known as the scissors position. With your partner flat on her back, her knees up and apart so that her legs are bent, move close to her and lie with your legs underneath hers. Intertwine your legs a little so that the nearest one to her is underneath and the furthest one from her is on top, with your genitals touching. She should be able to reach down and take your penis in her hands, inserting it into her.

Actually inserting the limp penis not only take practice; it may take a sense of humour too! But keep going; just as it was vital to learn to let your erection die away, so it is vital to know how to ease your penis into your partner's vagina, whatever state of erection it is in.

There is an exception to all this. If you know that you are seriously wary of penetration, then you may want to experiment with doing the direct opposite of what we have suggested, that is waiting until you are

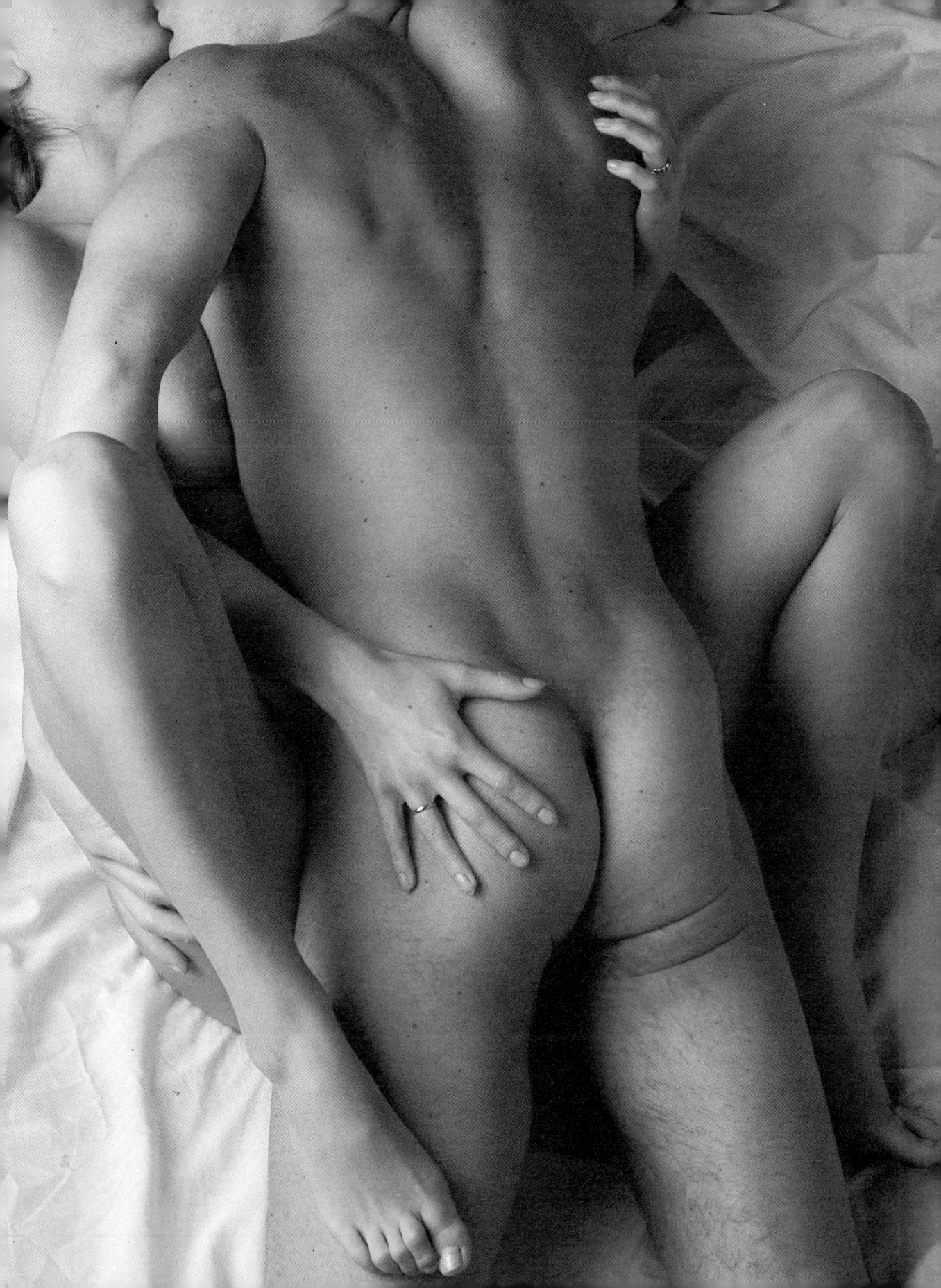

extremely aroused, and until your partner has excited you to a hard erection, and then entering her. If you do, then also use the woman-on-top position, which allows your partner to keep stimulating you as she inserts your penis.

ENTERING IN

STAGE 1

Once you have some degree of penetration, then lie still. Of course, the urge is to get it up at once, start thrusting and keep going until you come, particularly if your partner's vagina is warm and tight. But hang on in there; generations of Eastern love-makers have perfected this technique with similar self-discipline, so you can do it, too!

Keep eye contact with your partner; focus on the sensations you both feel. You might be surprised if she is actually feeling more with your limp penis inside her than with an erect one, simply because her vaginal muscles may have a chance to move more against it. You may also be surprised that, despite the fact that you are not thrusting, you are beginning to feel aroused; move slightly to create even more arousal.

STAGE 2

When you feel your erection harden – and this is the difficult part – withdraw immediately from your partner and move away from each other. As with all the other sexual explorations we suggest, the secret is to chart every stage by repeating it again and again, rather than continuing on to orgasm immediately erection strikes.

Once moved away, you need to let the arousal die, preferably until all stiffness has disappeared. What should you do in the meantime? Beside you is a partner who almost certainly is very aroused; one who, moreover, may need all the time and stimulation you can give her in order to really enjoy herself. So we are sure you can find something to do with your hands and mouth for the length of time it takes for you to become limp again – though, of course, if you find yourself becoming aroused by doing this, you may, for the course of these explorations, simply have to lie together holding hands!

Once limp, you can begin again, moving closer until your partner can insert your penis, lying still for as long as you can. Practise several times over the course of a few love-making sessions, and there will come a point where you can lie and simply enjoy the feelings, without needing to carry on and thrust. Some Eastern love-making techniques involve simply lying still, erection maintained, and letting the sensations come and go. The claim is that, even with no movement, they will eventually move towards orgasm – though we have yet to experience this one in practice!

STAGE 3

Once you can easily penetrate and lie still, you can start adding in more stimulation and learning what works for you both. To start with, perhaps you can move, just slightly. Kiss your partner, get her to move, as she likes, caress each other but, as always, stop as you feel the arousal start to build.

At this point, there is no need to pull out (unless you are mentally panicky about your erection lasting, in which case take the pressure off yourself by withdrawing completely). A pause of a few seconds or

Pleasure with Penetration

building it again may be all you need.

For this is the time when you are beginning really to learn about yourselves, when she is beginning to learn of the ways she can gain pleasure through intercourse – and you in turn are learning the other options available to you that may make intercourse an even more pleasurable, and certainly a more confident experience. To really build on gaining knowledge for both of you, you need to work together, at each moment checking out what you want; it is essential to keep communicating the whole time, in words, in sounds, in movements.

We would suggest that there are several ways in which you can play with the elements involved in intercourse.

● **Position.** There are six basic groups of sexual positions that you can experiment with: man on top such as is found in the missionary position; woman on top such as we suggested for ease of limp penis insertion; rear entry where you go into her vagina from behind; side by side such as the scissors position we suggested for ease of insertion; sitting, with either of you astride the other; standing, usually with her holding on to you.

The two positions we earlier suggested not only allow you to insert a limp penis and enhance erection quickly, they also give good equal control over what happens, allowing you to move in the plateau phase and let the pleasure come and go. In addition, they make it easy for you to relax, not get tired, and therefore last longer. The woman-on-top position was a favourite of both ancient Romans and Chinese because it increased control, and the African and Pacific peoples used it regularly before Christians arrived and enforced the 'man-on-top' missionary position, which they thought emphasized that sex was for procreation rather than pleasure.

Positions that can be good if you want to enhance your erection are the ones which give you a chance to penetrate her most deeply; these are usually man-on-top positions. The missionary position is a classic, particularly if you want to urge on your ejaculation, and you may want to experiment with where her legs need to be in order to give her some stimulation from your pubic bone. Do they need to be partially closed, giving you a lot of friction and her a closed vagina; do you need to put her legs over her shoulders so that you can penetrate deeply?

Positions that give you less arousal, and therefore allow you to stay in the plateau phase for longer are any that offer less stimulation. The missionary position is a total no-no, but side-to-side or facing each other are good because they allow slightly less penetration. Woman-on-top works well if your partner is controlled enough to stay absolutely still when you need her to, and also allows her easily to hold you back by using the squeeze technique we describe in Chapter 18.

If your partner needs direct stimulation in order to be aroused through intercourse, the woman-on-top positions we outlined are ideal. Move slowly and carefully, trying out different ways in which either of you might reach her clitoris: with fingers, with your pubic bone, with the whole of the hand or with a vibrator. If you want to try a different position, she could switch from squatting to kneeling or vice versa, or outstretch one leg. Let her also experiment with her body position here, leaning forward over you to kiss or caress your face, or back away from you with the weight on her hands, stretching upwards with her hands above her head, or even behind her back to show her breasts.

To guarantee direct clitoral stimulation in these positions, you have to place her hand or yours down between you, although, in some women, her squeezing her vagina together as you move can, as well as giving you extra sensation, give her what she needs. With her on her stomach, and you entering her from behind, she can rub against the bed or the sheets, or even get her hand down underneath to touch herself.

Equally, you may both be quite happy on occasion to choose a position that doesn't give your partner the stimulation she needs to orgasm, although this should only be an 'on occasion' thing. If intercourse is to be satisfying for her, then we feel she needs to be getting pleasure from it far more than fifty per cent of the time. If you have any doubt about this, check out how you would feel if, fifty per cent of the time you made love, she left you without an orgasm!

The final thing to remember about sexual position is that if you want to move back from the point of no return, shifting position can do it. You have to move very quickly, and often pulling out from your partner completely is the result – but it can be done!

- **Depth.** Whatever your position, you do have a choice how deeply you penetrate. Deep in will enhance your erection and often your pleasure; very shallow movements may be a totally different sensation which allows you to experiment. Eastern yogic sensuality teaches that alternating the two is best, counting perhaps one deep and then three shallow; then one deep and five shallow, followed by one deep and nine shallow. This pattern both keeps the interest up and allows arousal to develop.

Varying depth has two other built-in advantages; firstly, by stimulating the entrance to the vagina, you hit more of the sensitive nerves than the less-sensitive interior, which may be more exciting for your partner. Secondly, if you find that deep thrusts really arouse you, and want to hold back the pleasure and move further away from the point of no return, shift to shallow thrusts for a while until you feel able to go back to further pleasure.

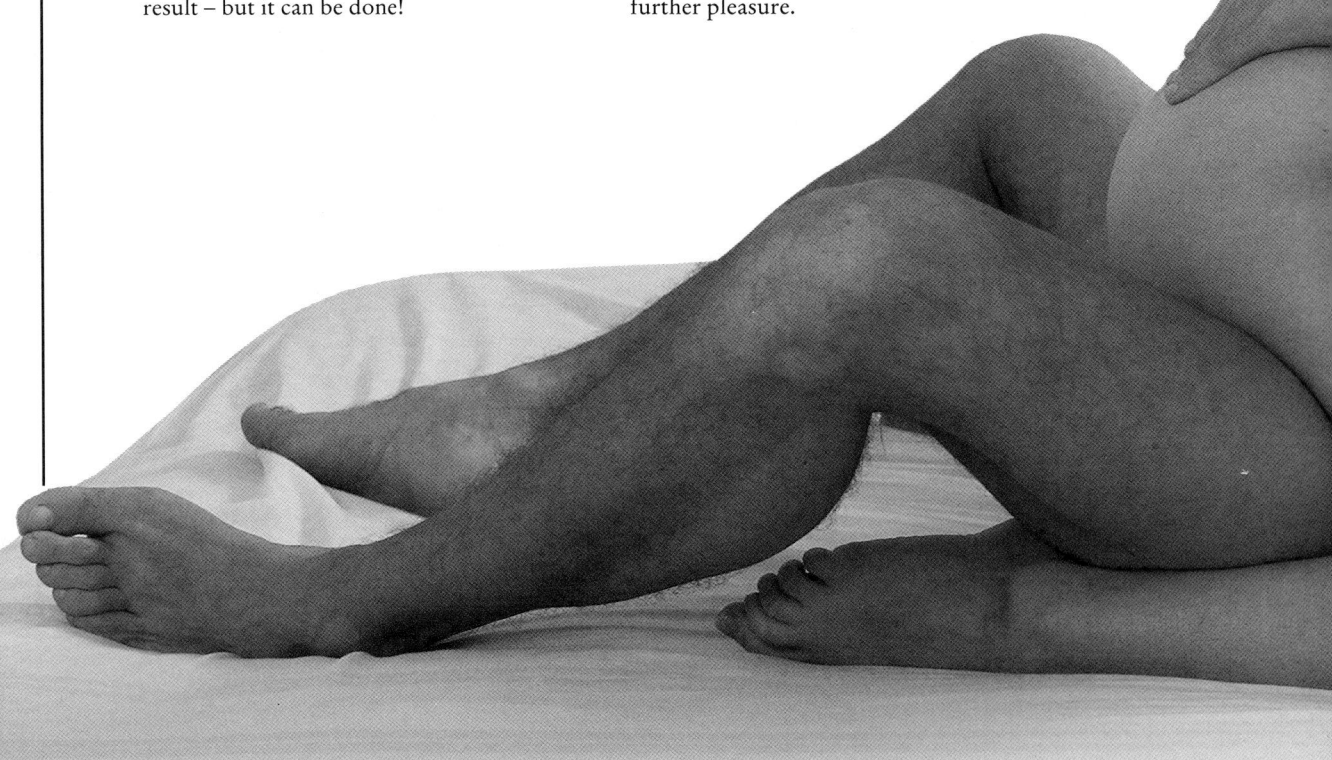

PLEASURE WITH PENETRATION

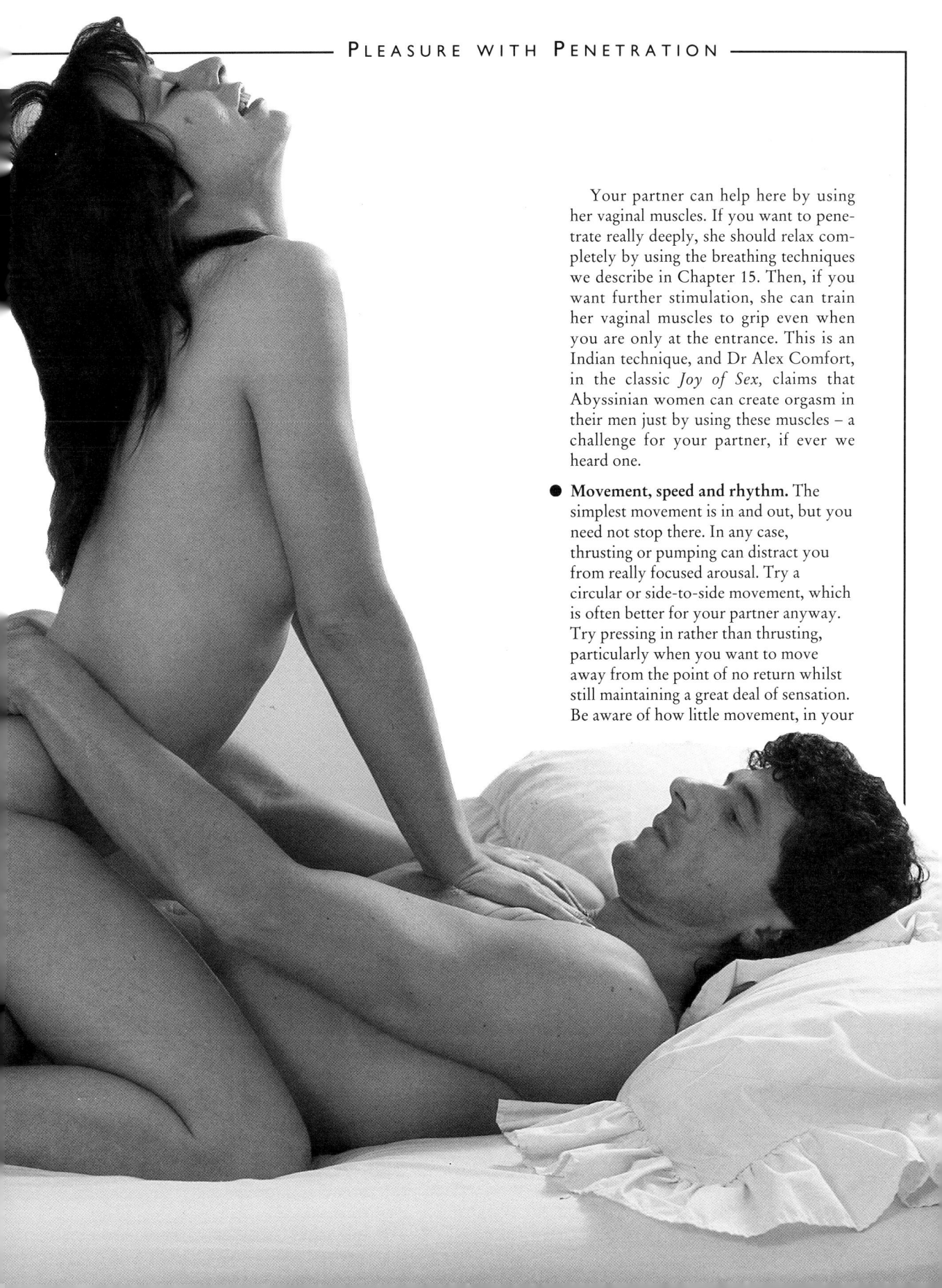

Your partner can help here by using her vaginal muscles. If you want to penetrate really deeply, she should relax completely by using the breathing techniques we describe in Chapter 15. Then, if you want further stimulation, she can train her vaginal muscles to grip even when you are only at the entrance. This is an Indian technique, and Dr Alex Comfort, in the classic *Joy of Sex,* claims that Abyssinian women can create orgasm in their men just by using these muscles – a challenge for your partner, if ever we heard one.

- **Movement, speed and rhythm.** The simplest movement is in and out, but you need not stop there. In any case, thrusting or pumping can distract you from really focused arousal. Try a circular or side-to-side movement, which is often better for your partner anyway. Try pressing in rather than thrusting, particularly when you want to move away from the point of no return whilst still maintaining a great deal of sensation. Be aware of how little movement, in your penis or in the whole of your body, you need in order to keep arousal going.

When it comes to speed and rhythm, you may be tempted to go more quickly and regularly as you near orgasm. But variations in both speed and rhythm are really useful tools in keeping you both hovering in the plateau phase without coming. If you learn to play with this, stopping completely, slowing down, speeding up, moving rhythmically for a while and then alternating with stop-start movements that allow desire to die, you can learn to pull back from the brink as you want to simply by varying the pace.

However you may find that what suits you in terms of speed and rhythm does not suit your partner, and that the quick regular thrusting that brings you to orgasm leaves her unstimulated, or conflicts with the kind of manual stimulation that she needs on her clitoris to bring her off. In either of these cases, you may want to alternate speeds, so that you get aroused so far, then switch speed and rhythm to suit her, gradually working up to a point where you are both near orgasm, in the way you would during mutual masturbation. Alternatively, go for her orgasm first with movements that suit her, then go for your own climax.

If you get into the habit of doing this, however, don't think that slow, steady intercourse is 'her' way of doing it and that quick, thrusting intercourse is 'your' way – this is blasphemy in Supervirility terms. Unless you can learn to have a range of speeds and rhythms that can vary in order to hold yourself in the plateau phase, you are missing the whole point of these explorations.

A final word. You can get to the point where you are so on the edge of coming that you can stop movement completely and still hover on the brink. Once you have done this a few times, experiment with how little movement and speed you need in order to tip over. Can your partner's internal movement alone do it; can your exhaled breath alone bring you to orgasm?

- **Adding sensation.** Finally, don't forget that in intercourse, as in all other aspects of love-making, the aim is to raise your ability to feel rather than pushing on immediately to orgasm.

So, while you are hovering in the plateau phase, also consider what else you and your partner can be doing to add sensation. Could you be kissing, reflecting penis movements with movements of your tongues? Could you touch her breasts, her ears, her neck or any of

SEXUAL TROUBLE-SHOOTING

As we have said before, though these are sexual-enhancement techniques, you may be using them with a particular sexual block in mind. If so, you may find these guidelines useful.

- You will find that, if desire has died for you both, rethinking your approach to intercourse will revitalize your love-making.

- The particular suggestions we make about limp penetration and stimulation-enhancement positions will make you far more secure about your erection and your ejaculation.

- The stop-start approach to intercourse will help with any premature ejaculation problems you may have.

- In particular, if your partner has not been getting satisfaction from penetration, these suggestions should help enormously in raising her desire and satisfaction.

Pleasure with Penetration

the other erogenous zones you know about? Could she be gripping your buttocks or running her nails down your back? Could you be using your voices to reflect the rhythm of your movement?

Could you be adding in fantasy, murmuring in each other's ears as you did during mutual masturbation, or running the 'video' of that fantasy in your heads as you move? Could you be using any of your repertoire of mental enhancement techniques to prolong the arousal of the moment?

You should by this time know that we are suggesting you practise with all these elements of intercourse, using several underlying principles to enhance pleasure and to raise your ability to feel it. These principles are:

- begin to arouse yourselves;

- stop or slow as soon as you get significant arousal;

- once arousal has died just slightly, begin again, adding in stimulation so that you can get more worked up;

- again, slow as soon as arousal begins to peak;

- when you are aware that you have reached the plateau phase, practise moving within it, getting as close as you can to orgasm, then letting desire die, adding in further stimulation, experiencing that, and again slowing as you reach the point of no return; and

- she may want to take more than one orgasm during this time.

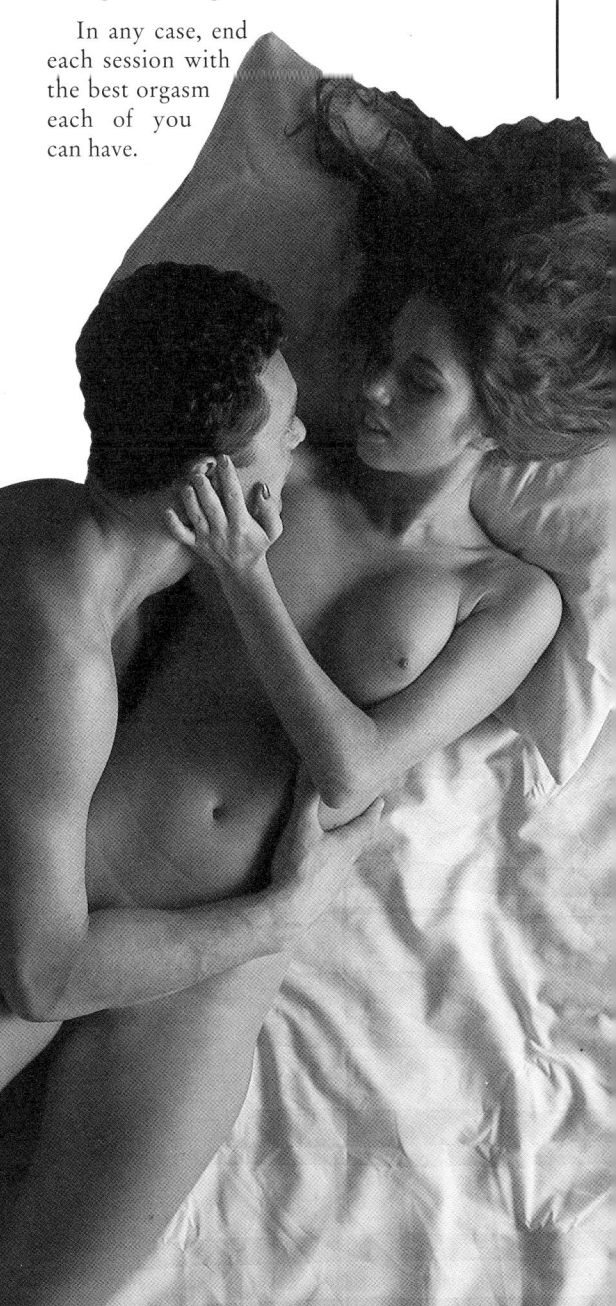

In any case, end each session with the best orgasm each of you can have.

Orgasm

For both you and your partner, the sensations of orgasm may vary from being 'like a sneeze' through to being, as the French say, 'a little death'.

For your partner, the central focus of her orgasm is situated in the clitoris. Stimulated either directly, or more rarely indirectly as your penis moves in and out of her vagina, this trigger mechanism sparks contractions of the muscles around the clitoris, in the vagina, abdomen, thighs, back – and can spread all over her body. She can orgasm once, or peak several times in a multiple orgasm.

For you, as we explained earlier, there is a two-stage process in a climax: emission and expulsion. As arousal peaks, a trigger mechanism comes into play which firstly makes your prostate gland and seminal vesicles contract, emptying semen into your urethra: this is the emission stage, which you will feel as the point of no return. Then, from your pelvis will come muscle contractions that propel that semen through the urethra and out through the penis: this is the expulsion stage, which you feel as orgasm, and see as ejaculation.

You will notice at once that there is a distinction between orgasm and emission, that the muscular contractions which form the pleasure of your orgasm are distinct from the release of semen. Orgasm and ejaculation are different; the ecstatic contractions that you feel are distinct from spreading your seed.

Orgasm without erection is possible, though we have known of its working in practice only rarely. If you want to try it, lie on your back with your legs drawn up and get your partner to put a lubricated finger inside your anus. Relax fully, while she massages the front wall of your back passage, about two or three inches in; this stimulates the prostate gland directly, and some men can orgasm like this very strongly. (Remind your partner to wash her fingers afterwards before touching your or her genitals.)

Ejaculation without orgasm is also possible, the muscular contractions simply never happening and the semen trickling out – quite a disappointment! Equally, you can orgasm without ejaculation; it can happen spontaneously, and many and varied communities around the world have also over the centuries encouraged it. People have found a great benefit to non-ejaculation where they want to promote (rather unreliable) natural birth control, where they believe that ejaculating weakens a man, or where they want intercourse to last longer.

This last possibility we would drop gently into your mind. In this book, we are not teaching the techniques of non-orgasm (which eventually spoils your response) nor are we attempting to teach the techniques of non-ejaculation, which often involves prolonged training in both mental control as well as physical. We do, however, offer some of the Eastern techniques for staving off orgasm later in this chapter. We are pointing out that failing to ejaculate is not the end of the world and, further, that not ejaculating for a while means that you can keep going for longer and have more pleasure. For, as time passes, ejaculation does become less and less necessary, and more and more likely to increase the refractory period to your next erection. And so it could be that, as time goes by and you are receiving pleasure from hovering in the plateau phase, you sometimes choose to postpone ejaculation this time, so that next time can be sooner rather than later.

Tipping Over the Edge

You are ready to come. You have perhaps hovered for a while in the plateau phase, but now you are ready. How can you and your partner make it happen? The key is, of course, to do more of what was already working so well. If you have integrated the lessons of Supervirility, you will have learned enough about your body to tell when you are nearly at the point of no return. So now increase the sensation without holding back.

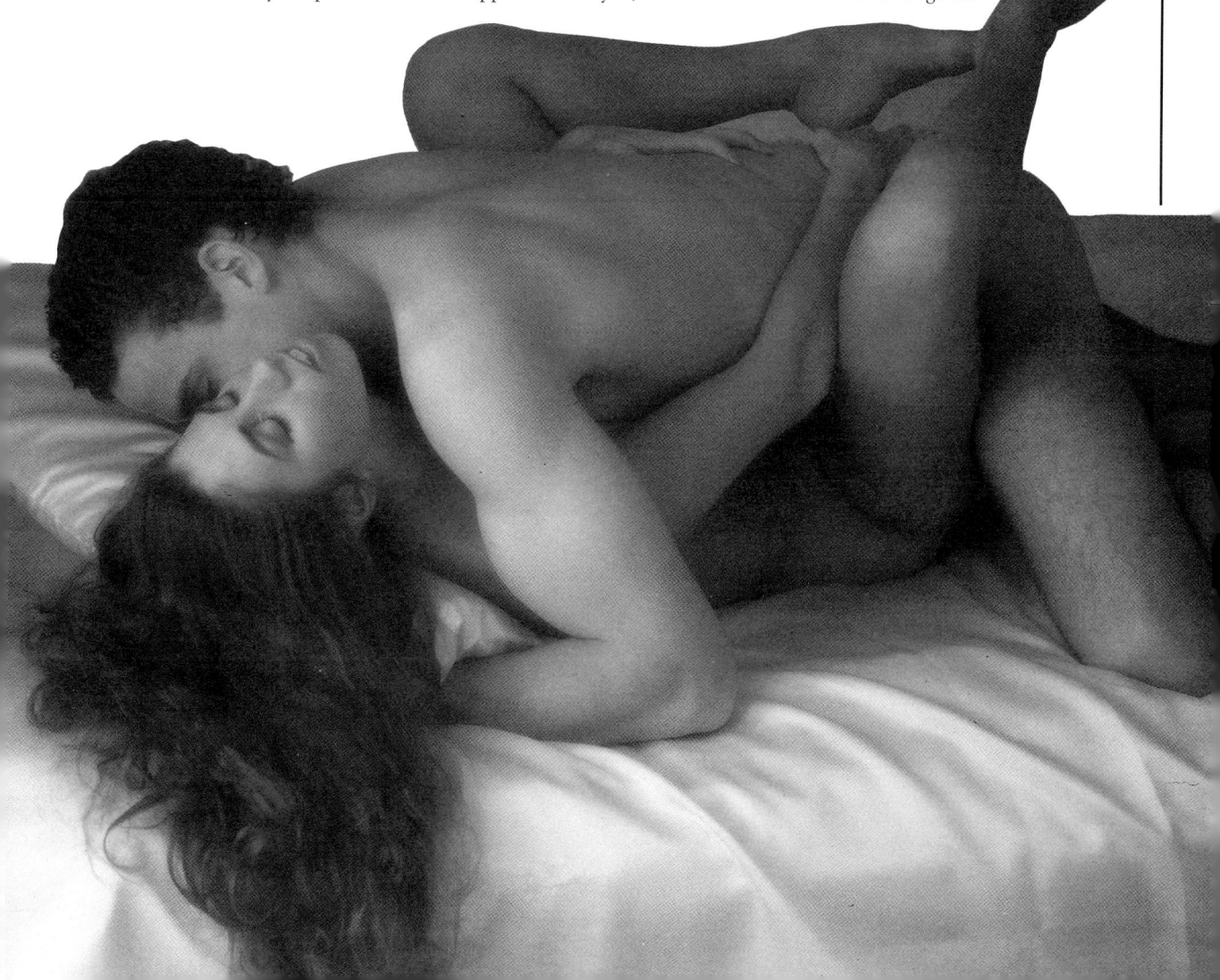

You can do this in a number of ways. Shift to a position that gives you maximum stimulation; move in a way that gives you the best possible depth; use a speed or a rhythm that creates the sensation you want. If moving your own fingers, bring all your skill to bear in doing just what is right; if your partner is using her hands or mouth, signal to her that now is the time to go for it. You may well need the urgency of her nails digging into you, or her body pressed hard against yours, vital extra sensory input to tip you over the edge.

Mentally, too, focus on the experience. Screen out all distractions; concentrate on what you are feeling, with no awareness at all of what is happening outside your body. Use sensory enhancement in whatever way is appropriate. If you are fantasizing, create in your mind the best orgasm ever, and if you are telling your partner what you are fantasizing, let your voice rise and take you with it.

Perhaps, as yet, your practice in these sexual explorations still leaves you a little uncertain about whether you will come. There is no urgency. If you can let arousal go, then it will come back, and you will learn to control it. However, if you do want to come immediately, and you get anxious as you reach the edge, then do two things simultaneously.

Firstly, relax as deeply as you possibly can, using the deep-breathing techniques we suggest. Secondly, concentrate as hard as you can, not on making yourself come, but on the sensations you are feeling at this moment. If your arousal begins to diminish, relax and concentrate on that; if it stays constant, relax and concentrate on that. Avoid any sense of trying to come, simply be aware of the sensations and relax. Tell yourself gently that you really deserve the pleasure you feel and that your partner wants you to feel pleasure; it is fine for you to come.

And, at the other end of the spectrum, balanced on the edge between coming and not coming, you can reach the point where, in the right position, with the right movement, aware only of the sensation, you can choose to let go – and with the slightest of movements, maybe even just a sigh, you can tumble over the edge into orgasm.

HOLDING BACK

The other alternative, of course, is that you feel yourself coming and you want to postpone that. You have not yet had enough pleasure.

As authors we are wary of the barrier approach to slowing down orgasm: sensation-reducing creams and sprays, obtainable from sex shops, or more than one condom worn to reduce sensation. The former, we find, can wear off at the crucial moment – and can make your partner's tongue go numb during oral sex! Both attempt to prolong pleasure at the expense of enhancing it; we feel that sex is about feeling as much as you can for as long as you can; we would rather you taught your body to slow down and experience the pleasure rather than placing barriers in its way.

The fact is that you already have the skills involved in delaying your orgasm; you only need to put them into practice. First, cut down all channels of arousal; slow down, stop moving, change position, get your partner to keep absolutely still. Stop the fantasy movie if you have one running in your mind. If you feel yourself nevertheless sliding, then get your partner to squeeze you (as described in Chapter 18).

Here, too, are some extra, more esoteric methods. A medieval Chinese sex manual suggests that you close your mouth and open your eyes wide; that you hold your breath gently; that you flood your mouth with saliva. Another method is to come out from her vagina, then press your penis hard against her pubic area; contracting your anus tightly is also said to work. Or you could try pressing your tongue against the roof of your mouth, just behind your upper front teeth, or sucking in your breath through a rolled-up tongue.

Incidentally, if you want to last longer and are happy that you can easily regain your erection once you have ejaculated, then beginning love-making with self or mutual masturbation can be excellent. You can then settle down to a pleasurable experience of prolonged stimulation, while your partner may well have caught up with you by having her first orgasm, and so be much more ready for her second.

HELPING HER ON

Of course, your partner's pleasure is as important to you as your own. So if you are ready to come, and she is still a long way from it, what are your options?

In the short term, if penetration is not important to your partner, then the easiest option is probably to come yourself, take a short break, and then start in again on her with hand or mouth. This has certain disadvantages: you may feel sleepy, or the break in attention may disrupt her arousal. And, if misused – you come, but then don't do anything for her – it can lead almost inevitably to her sexual disillusionment, with all the side-effects that that can cause.

But, if your partner likes intercourse mainly because you do, then she may be all too happy to complete intercourse and move on to stimulation that is more arousing for her. The key is to make sure that you both get what you want when you want it.

If your partner wants to come during penetration then the above won't be an acceptable option and you need to rethink how you can change what you are doing so that this happens. Of course there may be both mental and relationship reasons for this mismatch, which have nothing to do with sexual skill. But if a great deal of the time, your arousal speeds ahead of that of your partner, you need to look at what you are both doing in terms of technique. It is possible, by spending time arousing your partner, holding yourself back from coming, and being ultra-aware of what turns your partner on, to make sure that your arousal times are in parallel. Check that:

- you both have a clear idea of what turns her on: touch, sight, sound, smell, taste, position, hand touch, mouth masturbation, position of intercourse, extra stimulation on her clitoris, movement, speed, rhythm, fantasy, eye contact, sensory enhancement, using a vibrator;

- you have developed clear codes to signal where she is in her cycle: movement, sound, touch;

- you have made sure that your love-making has been wide ranging enough rather than simply beginning with intercourse. Try including early orgasms for her by hand or mouth, which often enables her to come more easily through penetration later on;

- you are giving her enough time to join you, by holding back sufficiently in the plateau phase; and

- you are clear about what she needs in order to tip over the edge from the plateau phase into orgasm: a touch, a sound, a feeling of real contact with you.

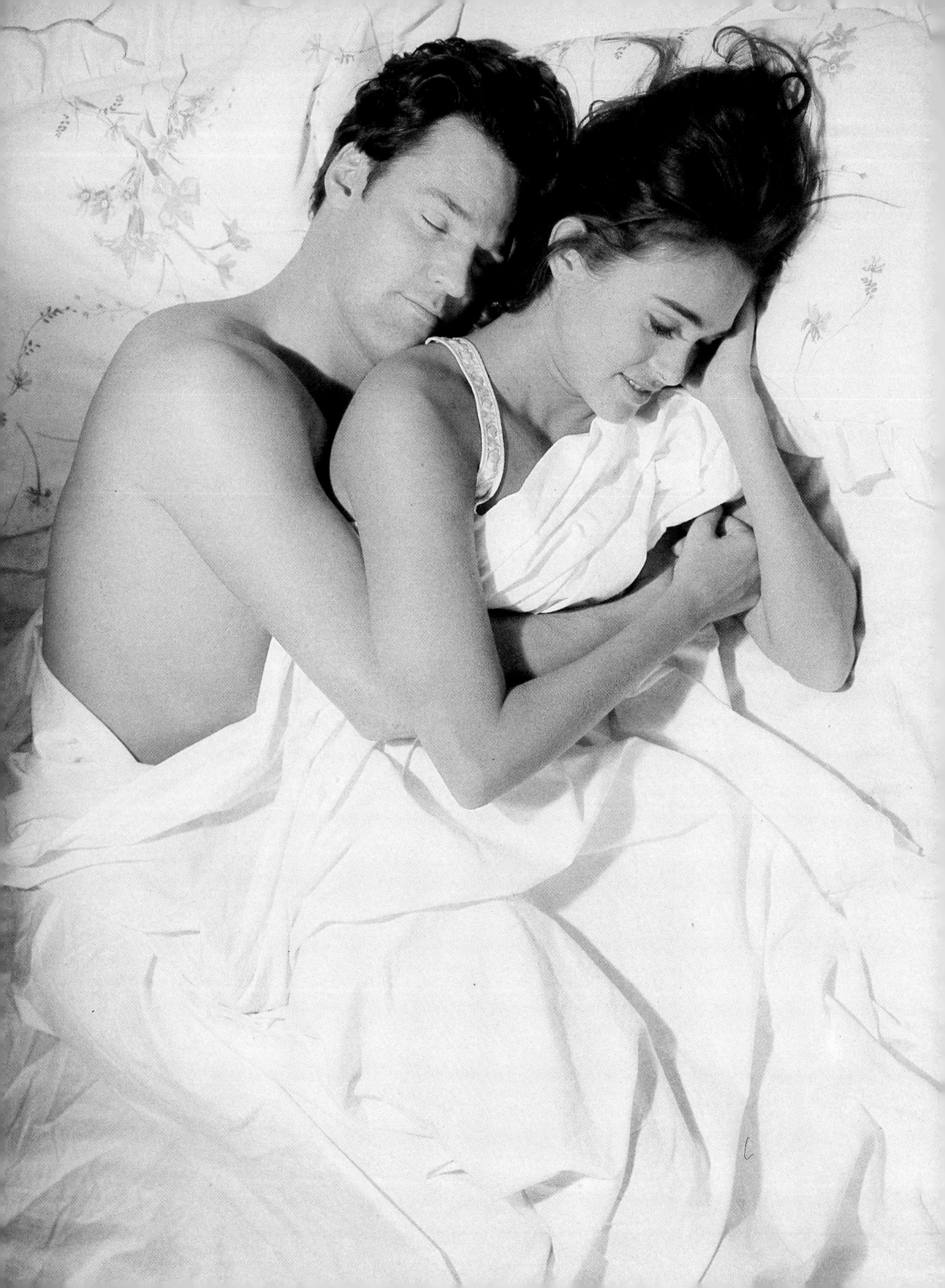

Coming Together

Supervirility techniques, which allow you much greater control, do allow you much more possibility of coming at the same time as your partner. If you both come up through arousal at the same rate, or can hold back while the other catches up; if you can end up synchronizing your pushes forward and your holding back; if you can signal to each other just as you are on the point of coming, and if you know just what it takes to tip each of you over the edge – then, in fact, you have a chance of coming together.

But Supervirility does not mean simultaneous orgasm. There are sometimes very good reasons for taking orgasms separately. It can be that one person wants simply to lie back and be ministered to – and we would suggest that such straightforward acceptance of pleasure is an essential part of a Supervirile love life. It can be that on occasion one of you wants a quickie and the other simply can't or doesn't want to keep up. There are times when one of you needs to come first – she to get really aroused in order to keep pace with you, or you to slow down in order to keep pace with her. On all these occasions, your best option is to come separately.

Afterwards

Love-making doesn't end when you come. For most of us, cuddling up with our partner in the security after pleasure is one of the best parts of love-making.

So make the most of it. You may feel incredibly sleepy, or incredibly active and outgoing. Your partner may feel the same as you or have a different response. Whatever your patterns of activity after orgasm, make sure you spend time with each other, whether in bed or pottering round the kitchen making coffee.

Talk and share what you feel. If you let out your emotions, that will give an extra dimension to what has just happened. You may think that, after several years together, you don't need to talk about your emotions, but even just a few words of intimacy can round off the experience. Confide something, share a concern or a celebration, an appreciation of your partner, or a hope for the future. Start talking about what you will do next time; without criticizing what just happened, plan even better things to do when next you come together.

It could be, of course, that the next time is very soon. For orgasm, with or without ejaculation, does not mean, at any age, that love-making has ended. First of all, your partner may well be ready for more orgasms; her refractory period is naturally far shorter than yours – and, with age and experience, that period may be considerably reduced from what it was when you first met!

Even if you yourself are not ready for an erection, remember that in good love-making an erection marks the middle of pleasure, not the start. There are a whole range of cuddling, stroking, pleasurable things you can do without even thinking about your penis. And the bottom line is that if, second time round, she comes and you do not even get an erection, then this is also a possibility.

So cycle back to the start: move through the range of options at your own pace. And do it all again.

LAST WORDS

Supervirility is for ever.

All the ideas in this book need to become an integral part of your life. It is not a question of getting healthy and then letting it slide, of adjusting your mental approach to sexuality for an instant, of making an effort with your relationship just this week, or trying the sexual explorations only for tonight.

Although initial effort in all these areas is vital, it is the long-term development in each area that will bring you most success – and most sexual happiness. As time passes, you will realize that the more you develop your Supervirility, the more you will want to do so; and the more you enhance your sexuality, the more you will see possibilities for enhancement. You will look back on what you used to feel and realize how far you have come; you will look forward to what you could feel, and see how far you could go.

Supervirility means seeing sex as:

- something which involves body, mind, relationship and sexual technique;
- an equal experience, where you both have easy and wonderful orgasms;
- the whole range of erotic preparation, self-arousal, mutual arousal and penetrative sex;
- pleasure, not performance; experience, not achievement; and
- continuous, ongoing learning in order to experience more and more pleasure.

We wish you luck in your sexual adventures. We wish you a lifetime of Supervirility.

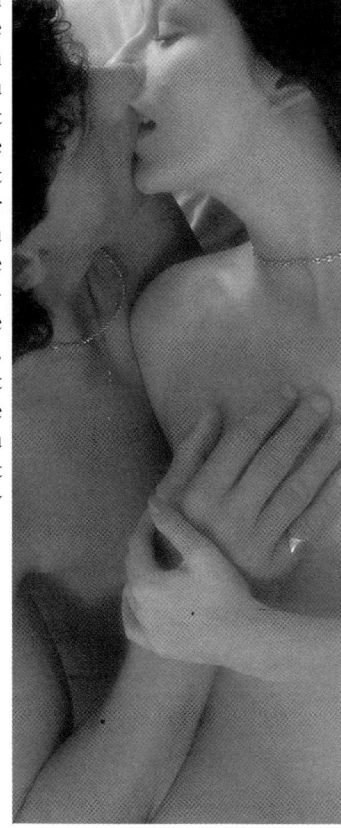

Appendix A
Getting Outside Help

Perhaps you feel that the only way to really boost your sexuality is to get outside help. If you do, this is not a sign that your relationship with your partner is breaking down. We ourselves have turned to counsellors to deal with temporary glitches in our relationship, or simply because we were 'only' happy, not ecstatic.

This appendix offers a brief guide to the possibilities in counselling for sexual issues, to what happens in a session, and to making counselling work for you. Sue Pallenburg, a therapist who specializes in working with individuals and couples, gave us particular support in compiling this section.

Possibilities

Kinds of counselling

● **Group work.** Joining a group of men who are concerned about the same issues as you are is a very effective way of developing your sexuality. These groups are usually contactable through personal-development organizations, magazines or networks. The personality development, support and debunking of sexual myths that you will find in such groups are worth their weight in gold.

Groups may be run on an equal or peer basis, where you each talk about your experiences. Alternatively, groups can be facilitated by a leader who has particular expertise on the topic being discussed. Facilitated groups can be more challenging, but those who prefer them say that they lead to more insight and understanding simply because there is leadership and structure. A group advertised as exploring sexual issues may involve some simple touching exercises or some talking about explicit sexual detail; the guideline here is that you never have to do anything you don't want to, but should be prepared to be attentive and not object if other men want to go into detail about their sex lives.

● **Co-counselling.** This reciprocal counselling method allows you to explore your own mental and emotional issues with the concerned attention of another person – in return for giving them attention while they explore their concerns. The theory is that although expert help is sometimes necessary, most of us can sort out our own mental blocks if given the chance. The essential basic training lasts approximately forty hours, over two weekends or a series of evenings.

While Co-counselling itself does not only cover sexuality, many subgroups within it offer particular help with the topic. Also, you will find a very open-minded attitude to sexuality within Co-counselling; about the only thing Co-counsellors won't accept is your trying to sort your sexual issues out by sleeping with another counsellor! Co-counselling isn't suitable if you are so distressed that you couldn't listen attentively to other people. So if you are currently in crisis, it is not the time to start Co-counselling – though once you've learned the skills, you will be able to use them to cope with crises.

We personally like co-counselling, not only because we are trained in it, but also because it seems a very democratic, self-empowering way of tackling blocks. The basic course is cheap; further counselling, workshops and peer group meetings are usually free. And whilst the training is not a professional one, it is of a very high standard. Co-counselling can be just as good or better than that you pay for.

● **Individual counselling.** This involves you working alone with a counsellor on issues. It tends to be relevant if one of you is very clear that a particular attitude or past event is spoiling personal enjoyment of sex – and that the other person, though affected by this problem, is not the root of it. This has to be the decision of the person involved – 'sending' your partner to counselling because you think they have a problem simply won't work. One particular, controversial way of working alone on sexual issues used usually with a single person, is sexual surrogacy. Here, a professional sexual partner makes love with a client in order to help them learn skill and technique. This provides an opportunity for one-way learning and confidence-building that does not normally exist in a relationship simply because you are mutually involved. A sexual surrogate will give all the attention to you, helping you through the problems in a professional way.

● **Couples counselling.** This kind of help involves both of you seeing a counsellor together. The first kind, relationship counselling, is most appropriate when issues stem from strong emotion within the relationship. Choose it if you are aware of relationship difficulties, or if you are fairly certain that your sexual knowledge and technique are sound, but you are still hitting blocks.

Sexual counselling offers all the resources that relationship counselling does, but focuses particularly on issues around sexuality, helping you to explore your idea of yourself as a sexual person, your love-making style and your body image. It is particularly useful for blocks that have arisen because one or both of you lacks knowledge or technique; where one of you has never really had a good sex life; where one of you has lost sexual confidence, perhaps after erectile difficulty or where there is a mismatch of sexual cycles or approaches.

Probably one of the most difficult issues around both couples and sexual counselling is for you both to agree to do it. One of you may feel strongly enough to undermine what is happening. Remember that such undermining comes about because the person is frightened of what will happen during counselling – this is true even if they appear to be angry rather than afraid. They may be wary that counselling will lead to a break-up, that it will be a statement that you are failing, or that someone else seeing your problems will be judging you. Sexual counselling may be more problematic here because it involves far more overt intimacy.

However, we can offer several reassurances. First, counselling in our experience rarely leads to a break-up unless one was already seriously on the cards. Secondly, attending counselling is far more likely to be a sign of commitment than of failure. Thirdly, no good counsellor would judge you for having a couples issue. They have seen many problems in their time, and are probably impressed that you are seeking help. However, these reassurances apart, if either you or your partner seriously doesn't want counselling, then you will do better to save your money.

Type of counsellor

Government-funded healthcare usually means you do not get to choose your counsellor, but with private counselling you have a choice. Do you want a counsellor of your own gender, so that you will feel more at ease? Does it matter if your counsellor is not of your race or culture? Would you prefer someone older than you or younger? Some people lay emphasis on a counsellor's qualifications, though we have found that some of the most effective counsellors are the least trained. The important thing is that you feel you can trust the person you work with, and that they are giving you what you need.

Time spent

Most counselling sessions last an hour, but some counsellors will work longer on a pro rata basis. Group work often lasts for hours; workshops can last for an evening or several days.

Commitment needed

Some psychoanalytic counsellors ask you to commit for several years; personally, we would say that, for sexual problems, this is longer than needed. Many humanistic counsellors working on issues that have begun in your childhood will expect to see you for several months. A standard marital or sex-counselling programme will last for between four to twenty weeks, with homework between each session. For brief counselling, suitable for curing trauma or a very specific issue, expect to spend not more than ten hours in counselling.

Costs

Costs vary enormously.

What Do You Do in Counselling?

Here we look at what actually happens as you move through the different activities involved.

You will begin all kinds of counselling with a chat about your goals and what you see as being the blocks to them. If you are in a group setting, then after that, you stay together as a group to talk through your issues. If you are in couples counselling, you will probably also be seen separately as individuals in order to check your past history. Be reassured that your answers will be confidential and a counsellor won't tell your partner without your permission – although if you tell a counsellor something that she thinks is vital to the issues, she may try to encourage you to confide in your partner.

In counselling of any kind, the counsellor will try to:
- help you work out what you want from your relationship;
- help you look back to the past and find out why you are hitting problems;
- reassure you about what you are doing right in your relationship;
- help you to see your partner's point of view;

- ask you to be really honest about what you like and dislike;
- encourage you to ask for what you want;
- help you learn that disagreement and argument are not the end of the world;
- make suggestions about how you could think, feel and act differently; and
- help you to work out ways of solving the problems that may crop up, in bed and out of it.

In couples counselling, the counsellor may also:

- support one or the other of you if they feel that the power balance in the relationship was uneven;
- support one or the other of you in order to help you to realize what is really happening in your relationship;
- encourage you to talk to each other about what you feel and think, particularly in areas you may not have checked out with each other; and
- encourage you to show emotion to each other.

Where the emphasis is on developing sexual skill rather than resolving emotions within the relationship (which is more likely to happen in 'sexual' rather than 'relationship' counselling) the counsellor may:

- make sure that you have all the sexual information you need;
- make sure you are not buying into sexual myths;
- help you build sexual self-esteem; and
- ask you not to have intercourse for a certain period in order to 'take the pressure off'.

Many forms of counselling ask you to do specific tasks outside the session. In particular, sexual counselling will set you specific sexual tasks to do at home, which not only allow you to re-contact your sensuality and relearn sexual skill, but also provide stimuli for the exploration that you do in the sessions. Whereas a relationship counsellor may suggest that you go home and spend more time together (or apart), a sexual counsellor may suggest that you go home and masturbate each other, try new positions or simply cuddle. Such tasks are often very similar to the ones we suggest in this book.

Often, just working through such a programme is enough to help you re-contact your desire once more or break down a block. But sometimes, emotional issues arise. So, if doing the homework makes you distressed, gets one of you angry, or lets you realize that you have gaps in your knowledge, the counsellor will welcome the opportunity to help you explore the distress, encourage you to show the anger, offer you information to fill in the knowledge gaps.

Don't think that these sexual tasks are forced on you. Most counsellors have a good idea of the kind of programme that is suitable, but they will adapt it carefully to suit your particular situation. If you feel that what a sexual counsellor is suggesting won't work for you, then he or she will do their best to respect that. The bottom line, however, is that most sexual counsellors will include specific sexuality tasks within the treatment they offer, and that you should expect that.

MAKING IT WORK

FINDING A COUNSELLOR

Your doctor will be able to provide you with a list of local counsellors or counselling agencies. Local counsellors, counselling groups or discussion groups on relevant issues often advertise in the telephone book; on the noticeboards of healthfood shops and cafés; through alternative health centres; through churches and community centres. Check when you contact them that they have experience in sexual and relationship work. In addition, there are nationwide organizations specializing in sexual and relationship counselling (see Appendix B).

DECIDING ON A COUNSELLOR

Your first contact with a counsellor will often be an initial phone call. It's usual not to go into details about your issue on the phone, but simply to check out basics such as whether a counsellor will offer the sort of approach you are looking for, when he or she can see you, the cost, and where the session will be held. Use this call also to check out whether you trust the counsellor and are happy to confide. If both you and your partner are going to counselling, it will be useful if each of you have a brief word with the counsellor so that you choose someone you both feel happy with.

Your first meeting will usually be your first session. You will need time to settle into your counsellor's way of working, particularly if this is your first experience of counselling. Even at this stage, however, you should not carry on if you feel uneasy or sense that you don't trust the other person.

HAVING DOUBTS

We hope that, in your counselling, you will get your needs met. What if you don't?

● **You or your partner aren't happy with the counsellor.** If neither of you is happy, however illogical your objections seem, leave and go elsewhere; trust is all in counselling. If just one of you isn't happy, this may be an attempt to stop the counselling for some reason totally unlinked with the quality of the counsellor; nevertheless it is that person's right to stop.

● **You or your partner aren't happy with the counselling.** This is slightly different. If you trust your counsellor, but the sessions are stirring things up, then stick with it for a while. Shakedowns are a natural part of any effective counselling. Inviting someone into your private sexual world and telling them your secrets may be difficult – one of our interviewees described it as 'exposing my wounds, baring my soul, feeling raw'. It can also be tricky accepting that outsiders are making suggestions and asking you to carry out tasks. If part of the counsellor's technique is to challenge one or the other of you, then this can feel threatening; stick with it and explore what difference this makes to your relationship. If one of you does drop out because of fear, don't pressure them back; you can carry on alone. If you find yourselves banding together against the therapist, then, equally, don't stop the sessions, as this could be a useful way of bringing you more into union with each other.

What if one of you does decide to stop? It is often possible for the other person to continue and get a great deal out of the sessions, although with sexual counselling this is less possible. The exercises that involve both of you are designed so that, although it may be possible for the one who is satisfied with the counselling to continue even if the other leaves, the counselling contract may have to be changed to adapt to the fact that sexual tasks can no longer be carried out as before.

CONCLUDING COUNSELLING

It is a good idea to work out with your counsellor, when you first meet him or her, what the goal of your counselling is. When you reach your goal in counselling, you can choose to stop, and many people do; you and your counsellor together will work to bring the sessions to a positive close. Conversely, many other people find that counselling is so helpful and enjoyable that they develop a new goal and carry on!

APPENDIX B
RESOURCES

RESOURCES IN THE UK

FOR FURTHER INFORMATION ON GENERAL HEALTH
Health Education Authority, Hamilton House, Mabledon Place, London WC1H 9TX (071-631 0930)

Institute for Complementary Medicine, 21 Portland Place, London W1N 3AF (071-636 9543)

FOR SUPPORT WITH ADDICTIONS
Action on Smoking and Health (ASH), 5-11 Mortimer Street, London W1N 7RH (071-637 9843)

Alcoholics Anonymous, PO Box 1, Stonebow House, Stonebow, York YO1 2NJ (0904 644026)

Narcotics Anonymous (NA), PO Box 704, London SW10 ORP (071-351 6794 or 6066)

FOR INFORMATION ON COUNSELLING GROUPS
Co-Counselling International, c/o Co-counselling Phoenix, 5 Victoria Road, Sheffield S10 2DJ (0742 686371)

Open Centre, 188 Old Street, London EC1 (071-549 9583)

University of Surrey, Human Potential Resources Centre, Guildford, Surrey GU2 5XH (0483 509191)

Redwood Association, 83 Fordwych Road, London NW2 3TL. Women-only sexuality groups

FOR INDIVIDUAL COUNSELLING AND SUPPORT
British Association for Counselling, 37A Sheep Street, Rugby, Warwickshire, CV21 3BX (0788 578328/9). Referrals throughout Great Britain

FOR RELATIONSHIP AND SEXUAL COUNSELLING
Association of Sexual and Marital Therapists, PO Box 62, Sheffield, S10 3TL. A letter and SAE will give you the names of therapists in your area

Brook Advisory Centres, 153A East Street, London SE17 2SD (071-708 1234)

Catholic Marriage Advisory Council, 1 Blythe Mews, Blythe Road, London W14 ONW (071-371 1341)

Family Planning Association, 27-35 Mortimer Street, London W1N 7RJ (071-636 7866)

Getting Help Outside

Institute of Family Therapy,
43 New Cavendish Street,
London W1M 7RG (071-935 1651)

Irish Family Planning Association,
36-7 Ormond Quay, Dublin 1
(010-353 1725061)

Jewish Marriage Guidance Council,
26 Frederick Street, Edinburgh EH2 2JR
(031-225 5006)

London Institute for the Study of Human Sexuality, 10 Warwick Road, Earl's Court, London SW5 9UH (071-373 0901)

Marriage Counselling Scotland, 26 Frederick Street, Edinburgh EH2 2JR (031-225 5006)

RELATE (National Marriage Guidance Council), Herbert Gray College, Little Church Street, Rugby, Warwickshire CV21 3AP (0788 573241) Will put you in touch with local counsellors

SPOD (Association to Aid the Sexual and Personal Relationship of People with a Disability), 286 Camden Road, London N7 OBJ (071-607 8851)

For contacting people quoted in the book

Dr Malcolm Carruthers, 101 Harley Street, London W1N 1DF (071-935 5651)
Hormone replacement therapy

Dr Martin Cole (DMCO), 40 School Road, Moseley, Birmingham B13 9SN (021-449 0892) Sexual counselling

Dr John Moran, 92 Harley Street, London (071-935 2182) Sexual counselling using papaverine.

Sue Pallenburg, 110 High Street, Sandridge, Herts AL5 9BY (0707-832503) Relationship and sexual counselling

Gabriele Stutz, 37 Peel Road, Wolverton, Milton Keynes MK12 5AX (0908-225051) Acupuncture

International Organizations

Australia

Australian Federation of Family Planning Associations, 70 George Street, Sydney, New South Wales 2000

National Marriage Guidance Council of Australia, 6 Morton Road, Burwood, Victoria 3125

Canada

The Canadian Association for Marriage and Family Therapy, 271 Russell Hill Road, Toronto, Ontario M4V 2TS

Planned Parenthood Federation of Canada, 151 Slater Street, Suite 2000, Ottawa, Ontario K1P 5H3

New Zealand

National Marriage Guidance Council of New Zealand, PO Box 2728, Wellington

New Zealand Family Planning Association, PO Box 6820, Newton, Auckland 1

USA

American Association of Marriage and Family Therapy, 1100 17th Street, NW, 10th Floor, Washington DC 20036

The American Association of Sex Educators, Counselors and Therapists (AASECT), 435 North Michigan Avenue, Suite 1717, Chicago, IL 60611

Association of Couples for Marriage Enrichment, Inc., PO Box 10596, Winston Salem, NC 27108

Institute of Marriage and Family Relations, 6116 Rolling Road, Suite 316, Springfield, VA 22152

Masters and Johnson Institute,
24 South Kings Highway, St Louis, MO 63108

Planned Parenthood Federation of America Inc., 810 Seventh Avenue, New York NY 10019

Appendix C

Recommended Reading

Cole, Dr Martin, and Windy Dryden. *Sex Problems*. Optima, 1989.

Comfort, Dr Alex. *The New Joy of Sex*. Mitchell Beazley, 1991.

Friday, Nancy. *The Secret Garden*. Quartet, 1979.

Friday, Nancy. *Women on Top: How Life Has Changed Women's Sexual Fantasies*. Arrow Books, 1992.

Hite, Shere. *The Hite Report*. Pandora, 1977.

Hite, Shere. *The Hite Report on Male Sexuality*. Macdonald Optima, 1978.

Grove-Stephensen, Ian, and Susan Quilliam. *The Best Counselling Guide*. Thorsons, 1991.

IPC Magazines. *Woman Report on Men*. Sphere, 1987.

Kinsey, Alfred. *Kinsey 1991 New Report on Sex*. Penguin Books, 1991.

Quilliam, Susan. *The Eternal Triangle*. Pan, 1989.

Stanway, Dr Andrew. *The Joy of Sexual Fantasy*. Headline, 1991.

Index

activity, declining, 8-11, 24-5, 105
acupuncture, 48
addictions, 35
affairs, 104-5
afterwards, relaxation/refractory period, 16, 24, 26 152
ageing, 11, 24-5, 72
AIDS, 45
alcohol, 15, 30-1, 32, 34, 35, 116
Alexander Technique, 49
anxiety, fear, 16, 90, 95
aphrodisiacs, 115-16
aromatherapy, 49
arousal, 23-4, 54, 86, 130-5; in women, 110, 111; see also erection
arteries, hardening of, 44
arthritis, 41
asking, 16, 75, 76, 95, 100
attractiveness, physical, 11, 36-8, 82
autogenic training, 72

baths, 119
beds, 115
bio feedback machines, 48
bladder problems, 41
blocks, primary, 12, 60
blood, 21-2, 41; high blood pressure, 41, 44
body, 12, 15, 20-7, 28, 36, 46; women's, 108-10
body language, 39
boredom, 58-9, 92, 123
brain, 22, 43
breathing, 117

cancer, 44
cardiac failure, heart attack, 41, 44
Carruthers, Dr Malcolm, 43-4, 51
cervix, 108
child-bearing, 85
chlamydia, 45
chocolate, 116
classes and courses, 48
climax, see orgasm
clitoris, 108, 148
clothes, see dress
cock ring, 47
cocoa, 30
coffee, 30
Cole, Dr Martin, 105
colon, spastic, 44
coming, see orgasm
communication, 99-100
condoms, 45, 115
contraception, 45, 115
conversation, talking, 38, 95, 117
Cowper's glands, 23
crabs, 45
crises, effect of, 90-1, 95

depression, 44, 72
desire, lust, 26, 57; lack of, 26, 57, 91-2
diabetes, 43
diet, see food
dildos, 138
'dirty', 59-60
disillusionment, 16, 90, 98
doctors, medicine, 15, 44, 48, 51
dress, clothes, 36-8; undressing, 119
drink, see alcohol; stimulants
drug treatment, 50-1
drugs, 31, 35

ejaculation, 24, 26-7, 131, 148; delayed, 26, 44, 79; premature, 26, 79
emotions, feelings, 16, 57-8, 65, 77, 84, 88, 95, 99
epilepsy, 44
erectile difficulty, impotence, 10, 15, 26, 41, 44, 78, 92-3, 130
erection, 16, 22, 23, 26, 66; aids to, 46-7, 50; early morning, 32; see also arousal
erogenous zones, 21, 22-3, 108
erotica, 103, 116
exercise, 15, 32-5, 48
experience, see past
eye contact, 39

failure spiral, 59, 92-3
fantasies, 116
fear, anxiety, 16, 90, 95
feelings, see emotions
first moves, initiating, 16, 114-17
food, 15, 29, 33-4, 35, 116
foreplay, 86, 111; see also arousal
future, looking forward to, 16, 95, 101

ginger, 116
ginseng, 116
glaucoma, 44
gonorrhoea, 45

hairstyle, 36
hang-ups, 79
heart attack, cardiac failure, 41, 44
help, need for, 13, 16, 35, 48
herbs, 116
herpes, 45
HIV, 45
homoeopathy, 49
hormones, 22, 43-4, 51

illness, 15, 40-5, 46
immune system, 45
impotence, see erectile difficulty
initiating, first moves, 16, 114-17
injuries, 15, 43
innovation, development, updating, 16, 79, 82, 100
intercourse, see penetration
intimacy zone, 76

kidney disease, 41-3
kissing, 123

letting go, 77
love, 88
lust, see desire

massage, 48, 119, 120
masturbation, 16, 124-9, 132-5, 136-9
mealtimes, 29
medicine, doctors, 15, 44, 48-51
meditation, 72
menopause, 85
mind, mental factors, 12-13, 54-63; see also anxiety; blocks; brain; depression; emotions; fantasies; myths; relaxation; stress
mismatching, 85-6, 111
Moran, Dr John, 50-1
multiple sclerosis, 43
muscle development, 44
myths, 15, 64-7, 125

nipples, 22
nonspecific urethritis, 45

operations, 15, 41, 43
oral sex, 133
orgasm, climax, coming, 11, 16, 24, 26-7, 66, 93, 110, 148-52
overdependency, 95, 97

painkillers, 44
papaverine, 50-1
parents, 55, 89, 95, 97
partners, relationships, 13, 16, 56, 65, 82-101, 102, 130-5, 136; see also women
past, experience, 15, 54-63, 82-4, 89, 95, 97

pelvic injuries, 43
penetration, intercourse, 16, 66, 111, 140-7
penile implant, 50
penile splint, 47
penis, 22-3, 41, 65, 66; see also erection
performance, over-rated, 66
personality, 74-9
Peymonies disease, 41
phobia, sexual, 12
piles, 41
plateau phase, 23-4, 26-27
pleasure, fear of, 60
pornography, 103
positions, 143-4
problem-solving, 95, 100-1
prostate gland, 23, 41
prostitutes, 103

rage, 90, 95, 98
relationships, see partners
relaxation, 16, 32, 48, 72, 117
relaxation/refractory period, see afterwards
religion, 56

scissors position, 140
sedatives, 44
self-esteem, 15, 75
seminal vesicles, 23
sensation enhancement, 129
sexually transmitted disease (STD), 45
Singer-Kaplan, Helen, 25
skin, 21; see also touch
sleep, 15, 32, 35, 44
smell, 38
smoking, 15, 31, 35
spectatoring, 58, 77
sperm, 23
spices, 116
spinal injuries, 43
steroids, 44
stimulants, 30
stress, 15, 68-72
success, problems with, 79
syphilis, 45

talking, conversation, 38, 95, 117
tea, 30
technique, sexual skill, 13, 14, 108
tension, 44, 48
testicles, 23
testosterone, 22, 43-4, 51
Thoburn, Marj, 88, 100
touch, 21, 39, 118-23
trauma, sexual, 15, 56, 63, 84-5
trichomoniasis, 45

ulcers, 44
undressing, 119
updating, see innovation

vacuum device, 47
vagina, 108
venous leak, 41
vibrator, 128-9
virginity, loss of, 84
vitamins, 30
voice, 38; see also talking

warts, genital, 45
washing, 38
weight, being overweight, 15, 29
women, 65, 66, 74; bodies, 108-12; see also partners
work, overwork, 15, 32

yoga, 48
yohimbine, 116

zinc, 30

160